17-95

TECHNIQUES OF
THREE-DIMENSIONAL
MAKEUP

TECHNIQUES OF
THREE-DIMENSIONAL
MAKEUP
BY LEE BAYGAN

WATSON-GUPTILL PUBLICATIONS
New York

This book is dedicated to
Charlie
and the
NBC Makeup Department

Paperback Edition 1988
A Backstage Book

Copyright © 1982 by Watson-Guptill Publications

First published 1982 in New York by Watson-Guptill Publications,
a division of Billboard Publications, Inc.,
1515 Broadway, New York, N.Y. 10036

Catalog Card Number: 82-1847

ISBN 0-8230-5260-5
ISBN 0-8230-5261-3 pbk.

Manufactured in U.S.A.

3 4 5 6 7 8 9 / 93

ACKNOWLEDGMENTS

I wish to thank John Caglione, Jr., who patiently sat for numerous hours under makeup during the photo sessions, and his colleagues, who pitched in during the classes to make the pieces and apply them, especially Barbara Kelly and Edward Jackson.

I am indebted to Dick Smith for his kindness in allowing me to use some of his formulas and include some examples of his makeup in our small gallery. My indebtedness also extends to Bob O'Bradovich and Carl Fullerton for their contributions and photographs. And a special thanks to Kevin Haney for his technical assistance and photographs.

CONTENTS

PREFACE

Prosthetics is an innovative makeup process that is now being used extensively in theater, television, and films. *Techniques of Three-Dimensional Makeup* came about as a result of a project in one of my classes in which we aged a twenty-year-old subject to forty, then to fifty-five, and finally to seventy-five. I realized that for this time span we had to employ all the available prosthetic techniques. Demonstrating such an aging process, then, seemed an effective way to teach the fundamentals of prosthetic makeup.

Most of the materials used in this book are readily obtainable, and the explanations accompanying the photographs are easy to understand and follow. I have also included discussions of certain problems and mistakes that you should be aware of so that you can avoid firsthand experience with them. The chapters are linked like a chain; you must study them in the proper sequence. Until prosthetics has become second nature to you, read each chapter carefully before you put the techniques described into practice. That way you'll know exactly what you will be doing and what you need to look up in other chapters. In fact, it is a good idea to review chapters as often as you can, because information introduced later is based on what went before. Eventually you will be able to bypass some of the technical details included for real beginners, but while you learn there are no shortcuts.

As you become more proficient, you will discover new materials that can be used, and like other professionals in the field you will approach your work more like a scientist or engineer than a makeup artist. Nevertheless, the basic techniques described in this book remain the same.

In addition to this book, however, you must have a working knowledge of sculpture. You also need a tremendous amount of concentration, and you must be neat, careful, and above all patient. Take notes on every formula you mix, every mistake you make, and every solution you discover to a problem. Finally, listen to and share your experiences with others. There is no room for selfishness and secrecy in this or in any other art form. You succeed in expanding your knowledge only by being open, discussing your work, and exchanging ideas with others.

Lee Baygan

PART ONE:
CASTING A FACE AND HANDS

MAKING A LIFE MASK

In order to design and create prosthetic pieces that an actor wears to look like someone else, or to portray an aged, deformed, beautiful, or ugly character, we must have the subject's life mask. It is taken directly from the subject's face by means of a special Prosthetic Grade Cream (P.G.C.) known as alginate. When mixed with water, alginate becomes like heavy paste. This substance is applied to the subject's face. When it dries, it forms a negative. A positive of this is made by filling the negative with plaster. It is over this plaster positive that the new face is modeled with clay as the basis for the prosthetic pieces.

This first chapter explains in detail, step by step, how the life mask is made. Before you begin, you must select all the materials you need and set up the work area. Make sure that the chair you are using is close enough to the table or counter that you can easily reach whatever you need.

MATERIALS AND EQUIPMENT

Complete information about the materials and equipment used in this book, as well as information about where to obtain them, can be found on pages 178–182. Here is a checklist for what you need to make a life mask:

Plastic drop sheet or large plastic garbage bag to cover the subject

Masking or Scotch tape

Hair brush, comb, hair spray, spray bottle of water, and corn syrup to flatten the subject's hair (avoid oily hair materials)

Bald cap of plastic or latex, or plastic wrap

Scissors to cut plaster bandages and trim the bald cap

Spirit gum or Plastic Adhesive 355 to glue the cap

Indelible pencil, felt pen, or marking pen

Petroleum jelly to cover the cap, eyebrows, and lashes

Mustache wax to cover beards and mustaches

Large rubber bowl containing premeasured P.G.C. (alginate)

Rubber spatula for mixing

Pitcher of premeasured water at 65° F. (18° C.) for alginate (before using, recheck and adjust the temperature)

Water or tank thermometer

Extra cup of water at the same temperature, just in case you need it

Five or six pieces of loosely woven burlap, 3 by 6 inches (7½ by 15 cm), to adhere the alginate to the plaster bandage (see page 21); or denture adhesive

Two rolls of 4-inch (10-cm)-wide plaster bandage, cut into four strips each of 8, 10, and 12 inches (20, 25½, and 30½ cm), for each section of the face

The shortest strips are for the jowls, neck, and mouth; the medium lengths are for the forehead and the sides of the face; the longest ones are to wrap from ear to ear over the nose. You also need a few small pieces to reinforce the nose horizontally and vertically. Stack these four strips in advance and use them together. You might need extra pieces to make the outer edges thicker, but the entire shell should not be more than four strips thick. The measurements, of course, will vary with the size of the subject's face, and you will need more if you include the entire head and/or the ears.

Bucket of warm water with a pinch of salt in it for plaster bandages (salt makes the plaster set faster)

Extra ¼ cup (59 ml) of alginate to fill the nostrils on the life mask; or wax

Krazy Glue

Extra brushes, spatulas, and towels

Spirit gum remover, alcohol, acetone, and isopropyl myristate to clean the subject's face

Shampoo in case the subject's hair needs washing after the cast is made

Soap and towel

Stopwatch or clock

For making the positive:

Makeshift cradle in which to rest the negative (see page 19)

Denture adhesive (Poli-Grip, Fixodent)

Japanese brushes for applying the first two layers of plaster

Small and large rubber bowls for plaster

Plaster-Hydrocal, Ultracal 30, or B-11

Wooden handle or aluminum rod, 7 inches (18 cm) long and 1 inch (25 mm) in diameter

Two strips of burlap for the ends of the handle

Metal spatula to smooth out the plaster

Surgical knife, plaster rasp, or surform tool to trim the mold

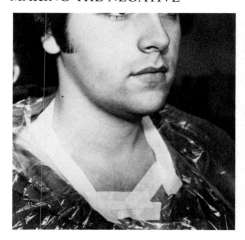

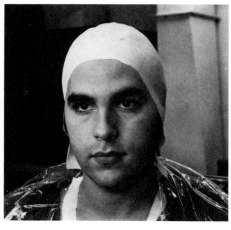

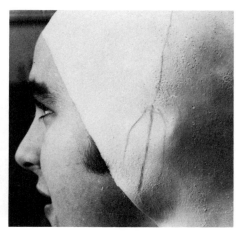

1. Have the subject sit in a comfortable chair, preferably one with an adjustable headrest. Cover his body with a plastic drop sheet and tape it around his neck with masking tape. If the cast is to extend below the neckline, tape the drop sheet at least 1 inch (25 mm) below the edge of the area you are going to include.

2. Comb the subject's hair back from his face, making it as flat as you can. Secure very long hair at the nape of the neck. To keep the subject's hair out of the way, place a bald cap comfortably on his head. (It is not necessary to use an expensive cap—a regular theatrical cap will do.) If the cap does not cover the temples and sideburns entirely, put a heavy coat of petroleum jelly on them. Instead of a bald cap you could use plastic wrap, kept tightly in place with Scotch tape.

3. Mark the cap around the ears and draw a line over the top of the head from one ear to the other.

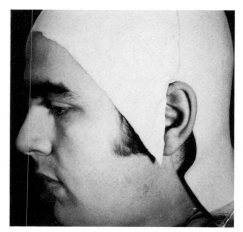

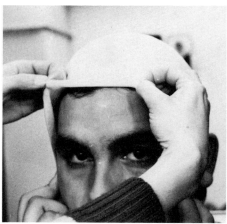

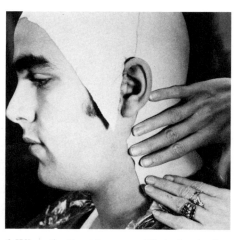

4. Cut the cap around the ears, but stop about ½ inch (13 mm) before you reach the tops. The cap will hug the ears when it is pulled behind them. (Some makeup artists mark and cut the ear holes out after the front and back have been glued.) If the ears are not to be included in the casting, do not cut the cap at the ears; simply cover them. You will have no trouble with undercuts (see Chapter Six).

5. Lift the front of the cap and apply spirit gum to the subject's forehead. When it is quite gummy, press the cap down until it holds.

6. When the front is secure, lift the back of the cap and glue it from side to side. If the subject has long hair secured in a ponytail, glue only the sides of the cap behind the ears.

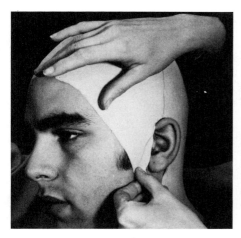

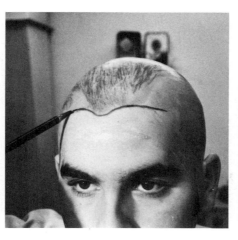

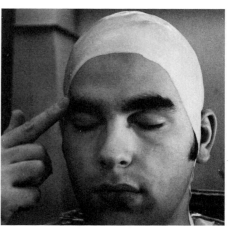

7. Glue the cap down over the sideburns. If some wrinkles appear at the temples, gently loosen the front of the cap and move it until the surface is smooth; then press it down again (the spirit gum will still be sticky).

8. Mark the subject's hairline with an indelible pencil or felt pen over the cap. This mark will be transferred to the casting material (alginate) and from there to the plaster positive. The line shows exactly where to finish the modeling of the forehead. Without it you might make a piece too low or too high for the subject. In this photograph the subject is wearing the plastic cap.

9. Rub petroleum jelly over the cap all the way to the line of demarcation and 1 inch (25 mm) or so beyond it. Apply petroleum jelly or mustache wax to the subject's eyelashes, eyebrows, sideburns, and other facial hair, such as a mustache. All this makes separation of the casting material easier. Be careful not to get any petroleum jelly on the subject's face, because the casting material will slide over it.

If the person whose face you are casting has a beard and/or mustache ½ inch (13 mm) or longer, neither petroleum jelly nor mustache wax will work—you won't be able to take the life mask off his face (though you might be successful if there is only a few days' growth). The solution, though time-consuming and difficult, especially when you have to clean the subject's face yourself, is to glue the beard and mustache down as flat as you can with spirit gum. When they are firmly down, cover them with a layer of mustache wax; then proceed with the casting. To clean, use acetone or alcohol mixed with myristate, or use Bob Kelly's spirit gum remover. Whichever you use, be extremely careful not to get it in the eyes or mouth. Stop the cleaning process often, especially when you are working around the mouth, because of the fumes.

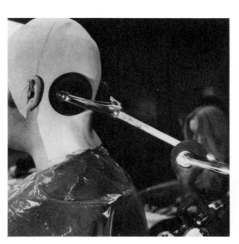

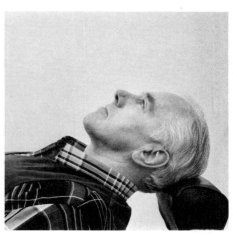

10. At this stage it is important that the subject be in a comfortable position. If the chair has an adjustable headrest, move it so that it keeps his head straight. If the subject's head is tilted upward or downward, the foam-latex pieces to be made later will not fit properly. (You cannot use the headrest if you are casting the whole head.)

11. Some makeup artists advocate casting a face or part of it with the subject lying flat. I do not recommend this because gravity can pull the muscles of the face out of shape and thus distort the life mask. Also, foam-latex appliances made from a face cast this way will not fit the subject when he is sitting up.

Before the next step, which is the application of the Prosthetic Grade Cream (P.G.C. or alginate), take a few minutes to explain to the subject exactly what you will be doing. He should be told what to expect during the process and how long it will take. He must breathe only through his nostrils, and he should let you know if he feels any discomfort. Find out if he has had a cast taken before and whether he is claustrophobic. If so, you must change your approach and cast the face section by section (see steps 20–23 on pages 23–24). During the application of alginate, keep explaining what you are doing in order to reassure the subject.

Mixing Alginate. If you are casting a face by yourself, it is a good idea to mix the entire batch of alginate in one bowl. How much is a batch? To start, use the manufacturer's recommendation: 2 scoops of powder to 1 vial of water (plastic scoops and a vial for measuring are included with each container of P.G.C.).

2 scoops powder = 17.7 grams
1 vial water = ¼ cup = 50 cc (ml)

A batch that is large enough for a small area of the face is:

8 scoops powder (70.8 grams)
4 vials water (1 cup or 200 cc)

You must multiply this formula for the area you need to cover: a face, a whole head, hands, or whatever. To make it simpler: 1 cup loosely packed powder to 1 cup water gives the right consistency. It is always best to measure both the alginate and the water.

If you keep the water temperature below 65° F. (18° C.), you can do the casting by yourself, but you must work quickly to finish before the alginate sets.

If you work with another person, divide the alginate into equal batches so that while you apply the first one your co-worker can mix the second. Working with someone else also requires exact timing. Test a small amount of alginate beforehand to find out exactly how long it takes to set and at what water temperature; you must also know how long it takes to mix the alginate in order to know how far in advance to have your co-worker begin the second batch.

Each makeup artist has his own method of working with alginate. You must bear in mind that the temperatures of the room, the water, and the subject's body, as well as the speed with which you work, will affect the result of the casting. The conditions for our demonstration were as follows: room temperature, 65° F. (18° C.); water temperature, 60° F. (16° C.); subject's body temperature, normal—98.6° F. (37° C.).

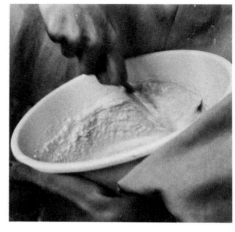

12. We mixed 210 grams of powder with 600 ml of water and beat the mixture. After the first 5 seconds of beating we added a dash or two more water. (When you have mixed alginate several times, you will be able to tell just when to add more water and how much.) Have an extra cup of water handy for this purpose. The alginate must be mixed until it is smooth and creamy. The mixing time is approximately 45 seconds. I have found that men beat this material harder and faster than women, so the time will vary. Be careful during the first few seconds of beating; until the powder and water are mixed, the powder is likely to fly all over the place.

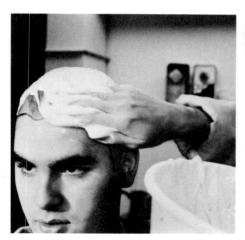

13. Using your hand, apply the alginate to the subject's face, beginning at the top of the head where you drew the line from ear to ear (step 3) and moving downward. Keep an eye on the stopwatch or clock, or have someone keep track of the time and let you know how much has passed. Or set timers to go off at intervals so that you know how much longer you have before the alginate sets.

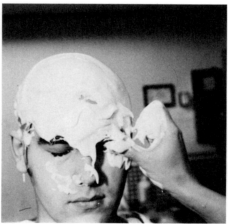

14. When you cover the subject's eyes, which should be closed, be especially careful to push the alginate into the inner corners and under the eyelashes with your fingertips. As you apply the alginate, make sure no air is trapped under it; use your hand and fingers like a spatula to follow the contours of the face.

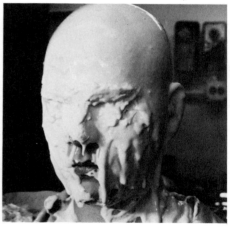

15. Cover the sides of the face, using a sweeping motion—don't pat the alginate on. Use enough pressure to get the alginate into all the lines and folds of the skin.

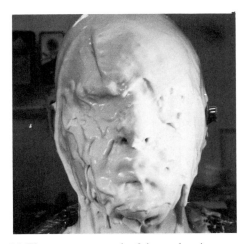

16. Then cover as much of the neck as is necessary. Next cover the mouth. Make sure the subject's mouth is closed, but not too tightly; you want to cast the normal, relaxed mouth. Finally, cover the nose, being extremely careful not to close the breathing passages. Don't let the alginate run; keep lifting it up over the face.

If you work quickly, you will be able to cover the entire face and neck with one batch of alginate. Try to make all the edges around the face, neck, eye sockets, and nose as thick as possible.

I have heard claims that it is possible to make separate, small batches of P.G.C. instead of one large one and cast the face slowly. Even if one batch sets, the others will adhere to it, and no line of separation will appear between the layers. Whether this really works can be determined only through experience and experimentation. The right way to proceed is the way that produces results.

After the alginate has set, which should take 3½ to 4 minutes, examine the surface. If there are any areas that are thinner than ¼ inch (6 mm), they must be repaired. Another layer of alginate will not adhere to the first one, so apply a coat of Krazy Glue to these thin places, make up a small batch of alginate, and cover the glue. This will hold until the job is completed. Be careful not to get any Krazy Glue on the skin.

The application and setting of the alginate in this demonstration took 4 minutes. Alginate will stick to your fingers, making its application more difficult as you proceed. It's a good idea to apply a thin coat of petroleum jelly to your fingers before you start. The alginate will still pile up on your fingers, but you or your co-worker can remove it easily and not lose any time.

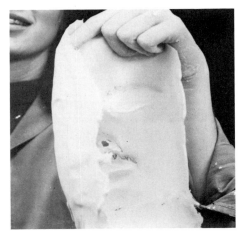

17. Even though the alginate has set, you cannot remove it from the subject's face because it is not a solid piece. If it is removed, it will lose its shape. You must therefore place a solid shell around it as a backing.

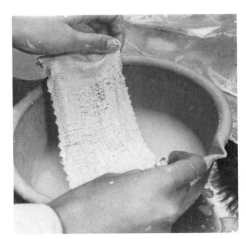

18. To make the backing, submerge strips of plaster bandages, four at a time, in a bucket of warm water that contains a pinch of salt. Leave them for only about 5 seconds.

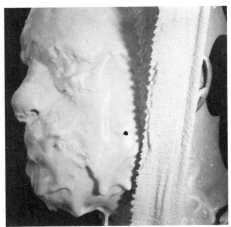

19. Squeeze most of the water out of the bandages and place them on top of the solidified alginate. Some makeup artists use three or four bandages at a time; others apply them singly. In either case, there should be a layer of four strips in thickness all over. Don't be afraid to press the bandages onto the lumps and folds of the alginate on the face. Make sure that all the pieces overlap and that the edges are thick.

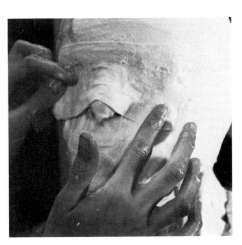

20. Next, with small pieces of moistened plaster bandage, go over the nose area horizontally.

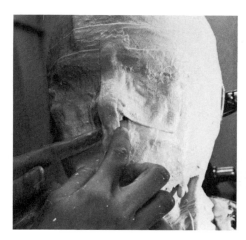

21. Then apply a bandage vertically. To do this, pinch the damp strip into a narrow ridge and place it over the nose between the nostrils; end it over the upper lip. Be careful not to cover the nostrils.

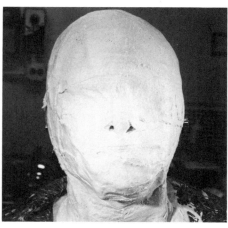

22. When you are finished, wait at least 10 or 15 minutes, or until the bandages are dry.

There are two ways of removing the life mask: one is to remove both pieces at the same time; the other is to remove the hard shell first, then the soft alginate. It is better to remove both at the same time; otherwise, it is difficult to replace them in the same place and position. Usually the positive comes out deformed.

In order to take both pieces off at the same time, have ready small pieces of loosely woven burlap about 6 by 3 inches (15 by 7½ cm). Before the alginate is set, press the burlap into it. Let it set; then apply the plaster bandages as usual. If the alginate has set by the time you are ready, or if you have no burlap or similar material handy, spread some denture adhesive over the alginate; then proceed with the plaster bandages.

In both cases the alginate and the plaster bandages will adhere together. You cannot use either of these techniques on the back of the head if you are casting the whole head; separation of the back would be impossible.

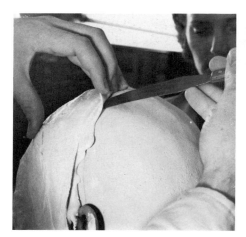

23. Before you remove the cast, whichever way you choose, have the subject move his facial muscles underneath it. This will separate it from his skin. He may feel some resistance on his eyelashes, eyebrows, sideburns, or mustache. Begin by separating the cast from the bald cap at the very top and near the ears. You may need to use a spatula to get started. It's a good idea to have the subject keep his face down over his lap, bending from the waist, while you do this.

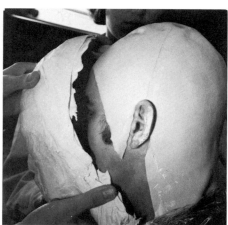

24. The life mask will come off easily into your hands.

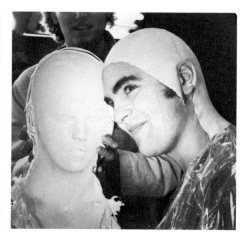

25. You have made a negative of the subject's face. (In photographs, most negatives appear to be positives.)

Examine the mask before you release the subject; if the impression is not perfect, you may have to repeat the entire process. A few air bubbles are not critical; they can be corrected after the positive is made.

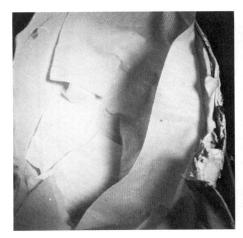

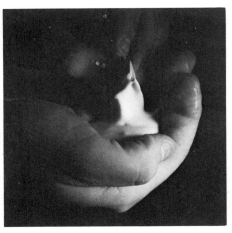

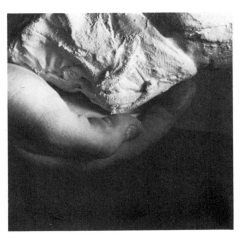

26. It is preferable to have someone else clean the subject's face and take off the bald cap while you continue, but if you must stop to do so yourself, place wet paper towels inside and around the edges of the life mask; otherwise it will begin to dry out, which in turn will cause the alginate to shrink. Do not put the mask under running water, which can damage the plaster bandages.

27. The negative of the life mask has two open nostrils that must be closed before plaster can be poured in to make the positive. To close them, you can insert small pieces of wax or modeling clay.

28. You can also mix a small amount of alginate in warm water, coat the palm of your hand with petroleum jelly, and pour the alginate into your hand. Very gently, from the outside, press the mixture into the nostrils of the mask. Be careful not to distort the tip of the nose as you do this. Let the alginate set before you remove your hand.

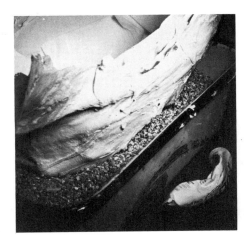

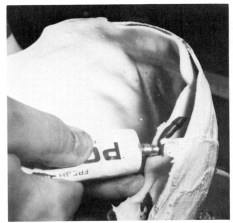

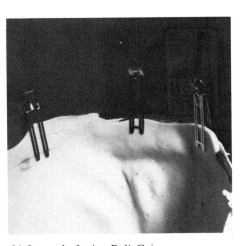

29. The entire mask must now rest in a cradle. There are no standard, ready-made ones, so you must improvise. We used an enamel basin filled with the kind of wood chips used for packing. You could also use sawdust, sand, or a rolled towel inside a pan that is large enough to hold the whole mask. Whatever you use must be high enough that there is no pressure on the tip of the nose.

30. Take all the wet paper towels out of the cast. If you have not used burlap or denture adhesive during the casting, squeeze a small amount of denture adhesive (such as Poli-Grip) between the outer shell and the inner piece. This keeps the inner edges from falling down or separating from the outer shell. Press the two sections together to spread the Poli-Grip; if it is uneven and lumpy, it can distort the mold.

31. Instead of using Poli-Grip, you can hold the outer and inner edges together with hair clips, as shown.

The mold is now ready to be used to make the plaster positive.

MAKING THE POSITIVE

By this time you should know how you will use the life mask, what size the prosthetic pieces will be, and how many you will need to make. Here we plan to age the subject gradually, from twenty to forty to fifty-five to seventy-five. For age forty we will need foam-latex pieces for the nasolabial folds. The pieces for age fifty-five will include the nasolabial folds, jowls, and neck combined, and separate pieces for the forehead, nose, and chin. For the final age of seventy-five, a single piece covering the entire face and neck will be used. Some makeup artists prefer to make even this stage a combination of several pieces rather than just one.

Once you know how the mask will be used, you will know whether the positive you are making now will need to go into the oven, so you can decide what kind of plaster should be used.

Choice of Plaster. All plaster expands to a certain degree as it sets. To get an accurate positive, you need plaster that expands very little. Some types can take more heat than others, and some crack sooner, de-

pending on how often they are used. The best material I can recommend is Ultrocal 30 or B-11, which is sold in 50-pound (22.7-kg) bags by U.S. Gypsum Company (see the materials list, page 178). As you become more proficient in prosthetics and experiment with different materials, you may find other plasters that work well. I do not recommend plaster of Paris, White Hydrocal, or the very expensive dental stones.

If you are planning to make more than one positive from the same negative, spray a coat of Polyester Parfilm inside the negative before you pour or brush on the plaster.

When separating the alginate, you must be extremely careful not to tear the plaster bandages or the alginate. When you separate the negative from the first positive, the outer shell will expand slightly; you must anticipate this and measure the opening with a measuring tape or calipers. You may find that the second and third positives are slightly shrunken, but it is a risk you must take. In such a case use Hydrocal, which sets faster, instead of Ultrocal 30.

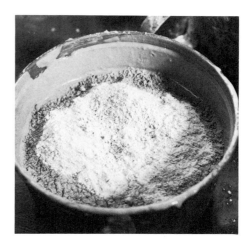

1. Pour a cupful of room-temperature water into a small plastic or rubber bowl. Using your fingers, gently sift in enough Ultracal 30 or B-11 plaster to cover the surface of the water. Let the water absorb the plaster. Mix with your fingers until it is smooth and creamy, like soft custard.

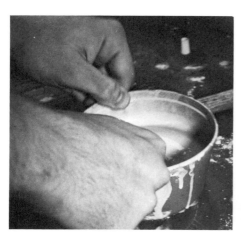

2. As you mix you will create a lot of small air bubbles in the plaster. To get rid of them, hold both sides of the bowl and gently hit or bounce it on the table—but not so hard that the plaster splatters.

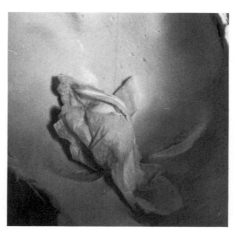

3. Put the plaster mixture aside and soak up any water inside the negative shell with a piece of tissue. Rinse your hands to remove all traces of plaster.

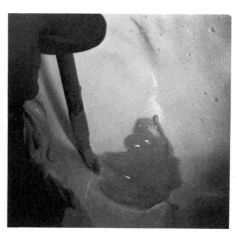

4. Begin painting the inside of the negative with plaster, using a large Japanese brush, until the plaster is ⅛ inch (3 mm) thick. Rinse the brush immediately afterward in clear water.

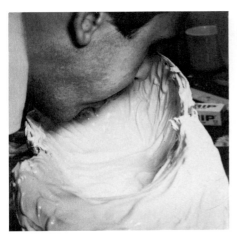

5. After each coat, get as close to the negative as possible and blow on it to spread the wet plaster and release trapped air bubbles.

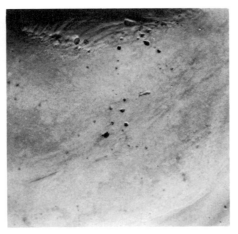

6. I have been asked if it is essential to brush on the plaster instead of pouring it. It isn't essential at this stage, but at times pouring has a tendency to create tiny holes on the surface of the positive; if these holes aren't eliminated, they will grab the foam latex and make it difficult to separate from the mold, resulting in torn pieces. You can eventually fill these holes, but it is good discipline to get used to brushing because it will help you later. It is absolutely essential to use a brush for the first couple of layers when you cast finished modeled pieces.

While the first layer of plaster is setting, mix another batch to a creamy consistency and get the air bubbles out. Do not apply this batch until the first layer is set. How can you tell? Notice that when you apply plaster it is very wet and shiny; when it is set, it loses its sheen and takes on a dull, satiny finish. If you wait longer, the plaster dries totally and slight pressure may crack it. One of the problems with Ultrocal 30 is that it gets hard suddenly. You must get acquainted with its action, which has a lot to do with the temperature of the water and the consistency of the mixture, by testing and timing.

When you mix more than one batch of plaster, try to make the consistencies of the mixtures as nearly alike as you can. You will probably waste a great deal of plaster at first because you don't know how much is needed for a certain amount of water or the size of the area to be cast. The best way to conserve materials is to mix small batches, and for future reference to keep a record of the amounts of water and plaster you use to obtain different consistencies.

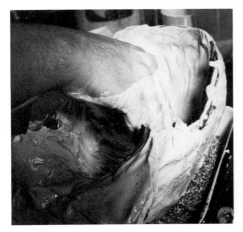

7. While the first couple of layers of plaster are setting, mix a larger amount of plaster in a larger bowl, using about 2 or 3 cups (474 to 711 ml) of water. As before, pour the water into the bowl first and sift through your fingers enough plaster to cover the surface. Let the water absorb the plaster; then mix it with your fingers until it is creamy-smooth. Make sure there are no air bubbles trapped under the surface. With your hand apply the plaster to the inside of the mold before the first two layers are totally dry. Build up the inner part of the mold to a thickness of ½ inch (13 mm).

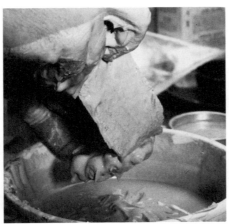

8. Depending on how many times you will have to place this mold in the oven, you may need to reinforce it to prevent cracking. For this mix a batch of plaster, cut short strips of burlap, and soak each strip in plaster. Instead of burlap you can use angel hair, but you must wear a pair of rubber gloves to keep the glass fibers from getting into your hands.

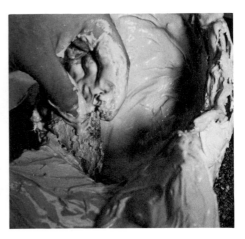

9. Remove each strip from the plaster and, without squeezing it out, place it against the inner wall of the mold. Press gently to hold it in place. A couple of layers of burlap all around should create good reinforcement. The strips should overlap for best results. Go over the entire inner surface with more plaster, until the wall is an even 1½ to 2 inches (4 to 5 cm) thick, depending on the size of the mold.

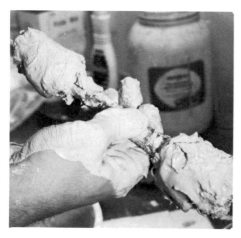

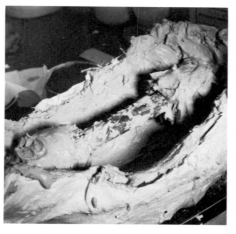

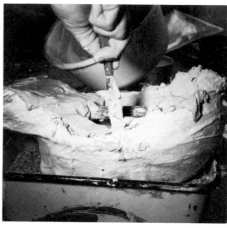

10. To be able to get the positive out of the negative later on, you need a wooden handle inside the mold. There must be enough space for the handle and for you to wrap your fingers around it. Use a wooden handle or aluminum rod 6 to 7 inches (15 to 18 cm) long (the size depends on the size of the mold) and at least 1 inch (25 mm) in diameter. Wrap a strip of burlap soaked in plaster on each end.

11. Place the handle in the center of the mold and secure it with plaster at each end.

12. When the handle is in place, add plaster under, around, and over it.

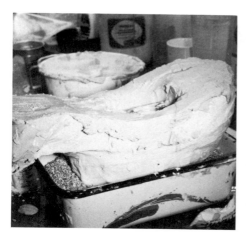

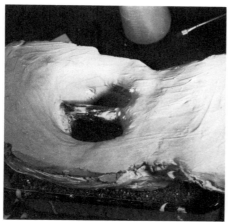

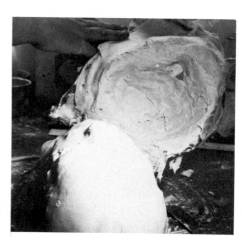

13. Smooth the surface of the mold with a spatula or your fingers and allow the plaster to dry.

14. Before the plaster is totally dry, trim and remove unnecessary pieces with a surgical knife. The plaster must go through some chemical changes before it is ready. It will get hot, then cold. The best time to separate the positive and negative is when the heat has subsided but the plaster is not yet cold. If it gets too cold or if you leave the molds to be separated later, the plaster begins to absorb moisture from the alginate. When that happens, separation becomes difficult and you might be forced to use a knife or spatula to separate the molds, risking damage to the positive.

15. Turn the mold over and remove the plaster bandages; if necessary, use a surgical knife or a razor blade to cut them off.

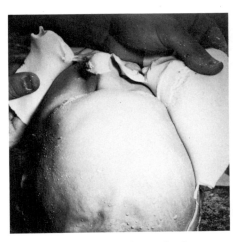

16. Remove the alginate by tearing it.

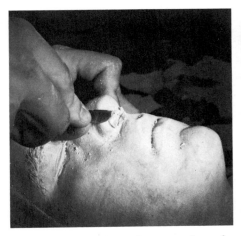

17. Trim and smooth out the outer edges of the mold. Cut off any lumps caused by air bubbles with a surgical knife.

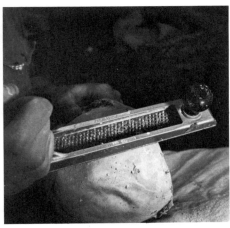

18. Smooth out the line of demarcation created by the bald cap with a rasp or sur-form tool, and fill in any holes on the surface caused by air bubbles.

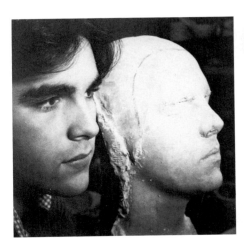

19. The life mask is now ready for modeling.

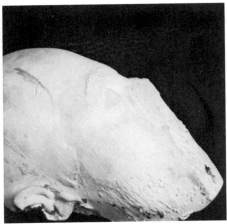

20. In the course of one project we came across a subject who claimed he did not suffer from claustrophobia. As we covered his face and mouth, however, he became panic-stricken, and we had no choice but to remove the alginate from his mouth and nose. (At times you have to remove the entire facial covering.) He calmed down while we added the plaster bandages and removed the life mask without nose and mouth. Then we made a Hydrocal positive.

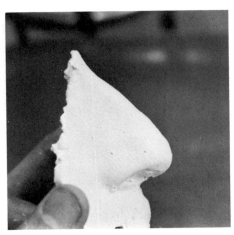

21. We took a separate impression of his nose while he breathed through his mouth.

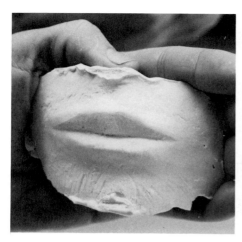

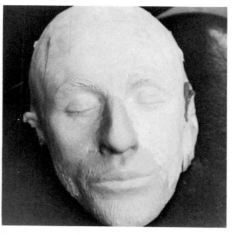

22. We also took the impression of his mouth while he breathed through his nostrils.

23. We used these two separate pieces as a guide to complete the life mask with modeling clay. The next step was taking the negative of this with another batch of alginate and making a positive of it with Ultrocal 30.

If the original life mask (positive) is made of Hydrocal and you need to make another life mask from it:

1. Place the life mask on a board over the worktable. If there are any openings or gaps between it and the board, fill and smooth them with water clay. You can take care of obvious undercuts (see Chapter Six) at the same time.

2. Apply a coat of cap material (see the complete materials list on page 178) all over the life mask and let it dry.

3. Following the procedure explained in this chapter, mix the alginate and apply it all over the life mask. Since you do not have to worry about a live subject's being able to breathe, you can make the alginate thicker and work faster, decreasing the chances of its running.

4. When it is set, loosen the alginate from the plaster. (A live subject would move his muscles at this point.)

5. Apply the plaster bandages. Allow them to dry; remove the whole mask carefully.

Before making the positive, measure the original life mask from temple to temple, jaw to jaw, and across the neck with calipers. Check these measurements against those of the negative you have just made to be sure they are the same. Sometimes the negative gets stretched when the plaster bandages and alginate are being removed. If so, the shape of the next positive will differ.

CHAPTER TWO

BREAKDOWN OF THE LIFE MASK

When it is necessary to age a character gradually, you can use high-lights and shadows or liquid latex to get the right effect up to a certain age. But eventually you must resort to three-dimensional makeup, known as prosthetics, to create falling jowls, bags under eyes, double chins, and other signs of age. For this the life mask must be broken down into its components: nose, chin, forehead, the sides of the face, neck, and double chin combined.

You may wonder why those sections were not cast directly from the subject's face while we were casting the whole face. It can be done. If you decide to do it this way, the technique is exactly the same as for casting the whole face, except that you cast one section at a time. In that case you really need a couple of people to help you. For the purposes of this book, we decided to cast the pieces from the original mold. That gives us more time to plan the prosthetic pieces.

MATERIALS AND EQUIPMENT

Subject's life mask in Ultrocal 30, B-11, or Hydrocal

Pencil

Modeling clay or water clay

Surgical knife

Metal spatula

Ruler

Pitcher of water

Measuring cups

Two rubber or plastic bowls

Alginate

Rubber spatula

Rubber matting

Masking tape

Petroleum jelly

Wire cloth

Wire cutters

Pliers

Plaster (B-11 or Ultracal 30)

Electric or hand drill

¼-inch (6-mm) drill bit and ¾-inch (19-mm) router bit

Scissors

Celastic

Acetone

¾-inch (19-mm) brushes

Japanese brushes

Plaster rasp

THE NOSE: MAKING A NEGATIVE

There is only one easy way to duplicate the nose from a life mask: with alginate.

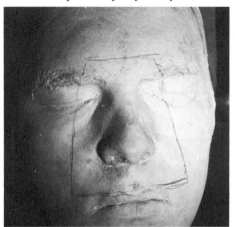

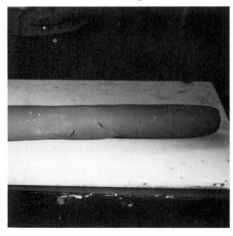

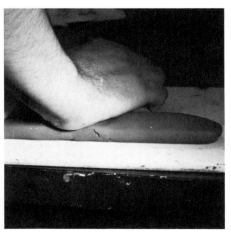

1. Place the life mask on a piece of smooth board, wood or Plexiglas, on top of your worktable. (With the extra board you can move the mold in any direction you want for easier handling.) Outline the nose area with pencil, about ½ inch (13 mm) from the nostrils and down to the upper lip.

2. Roll some used modeling clay or water clay into a log. Shape the clay until you have a smooth roll about 1½ inches (4 cm) in diameter.

3. Press it down with your hands to make a flat piece about 2½ inches (6 cm) wide by ½ inch (13 mm) thick.

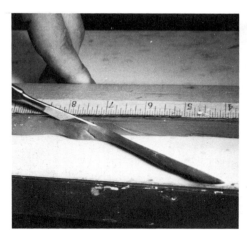

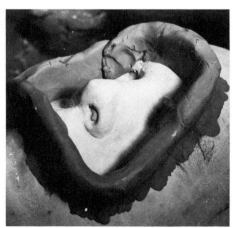

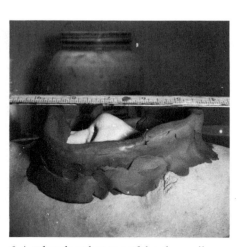

4. Put a ruler on top of the clay, or place the clay at the very edge of the table, and with a spatula or surgical knife trim the edges straight on each side.

5. Lift the clay from the table and place it on edge at the outer side of the pencil mark on the plaster mold. Press it down to make it stick. If necessary, anchor it from the back with more clay. The clay wall has to be long enough to go all the way around the nose on the line you made in step 1. If the strip falls short, make another and press the two together to connect them. The inside of this wall should be stuck firmly to the plaster at the edge of the pencil mark so that no liquid can get under it. You can use a modeling tool to achieve this result.

6. A ruler placed on top of the clay wall should have about ½ inch (13 mm) of space between it and the tip of the nose.

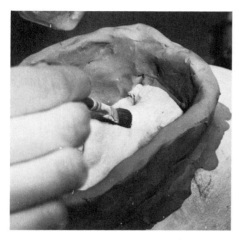

7. Apply petroleum jelly to the plaster mold inside the wall, using a brush.

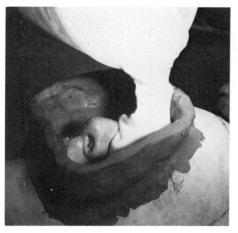

8. Mix a small batch of alginate in water at about 70° F. (21° C.) and pour it inside the clay wall. The alginate should be fluid enough that it can be easily poured and spread. Pour it from one side and let it spread until it reaches the top of the clay wall. This way no air bubbles will be trapped.

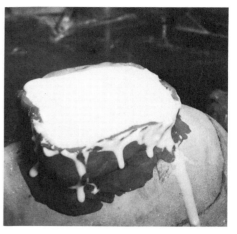

9. Allow the alginate to set. Because of its thickness, there is no need for a plaster backing.

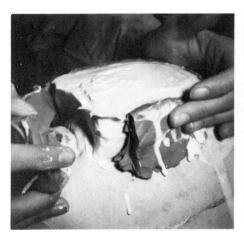

10. Remove the clay wall.

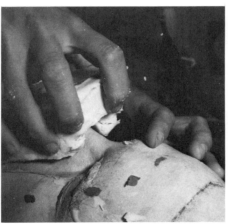

11. Remove the alginate by first lifting the bridge side of the nose, then the rest. If you remove the alginate from the tip of the nose you might damage the nostrils.

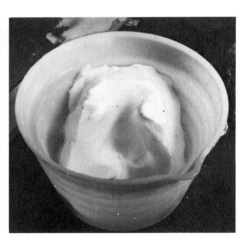

12. The negative of the subject's nose is completed. Place it in a bowl of water while you mix the plaster to make the positive.

THE NOSE: MAKING A POSITIVE

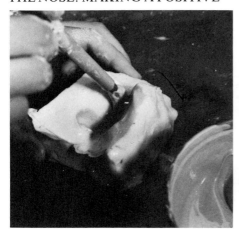

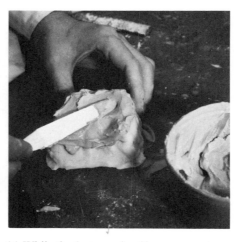

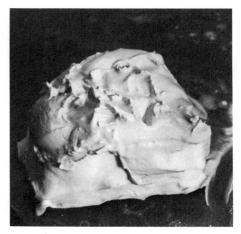

13. Mix a very small amount of plaster (Ultracal 30 or B-11) until it is smooth and creamy, without air bubbles. Take the negative out of the water, dry the inside of it with tissues, and paint the plaster inside it with a Japanese brush. Always let the first layer set before applying the second, and always rinse the brush after each use.

14. While the first couple of layers are setting, mix another batch of plaster and fill the nose, either by gently pouring it from one side or by using a metal spatula to build it up.

15. Slowly build up the plaster to about 1 inch (25 mm) above the surface of the alginate, keeping the surface as *uneven* as you can. (An uneven surface will grip the plaster block better.) While the plaster sets, prepare the materials you need for the next step.

SETTING THE NOSE IN A BLOCK

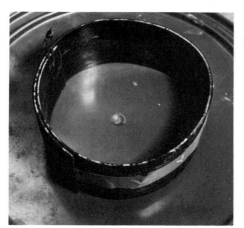

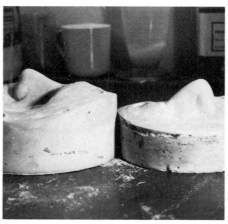

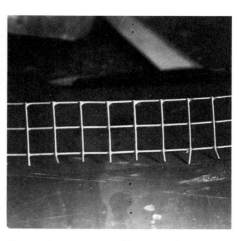

16. You need to anchor the piece in a block so that it can be used as a mold. Create a circle about 6 inches (15 cm) in diameter with a strip of rubber matting about 3 to 4 inches (7½ to 10 cm) wide and 24 inches (61 cm) long or longer. Secure it by wrapping a piece of masking tape around it. It is not a bad idea to use a hair clip to fasten the inner end of the strip. Rub petroleum jelly under the rubber circle for easy removal, especially if you are using a wooden board under the mold.

17. It is necessary to use wire reinforcement if you know you will use the mold more than three or four times or if you plan to save it for later use. Otherwise, you can save a lot of plaster by not using the reinforcement. In this photograph you see two molds that have been set in the same way. The one on the right is thinner than the one on the left, because the latter has a wire reinforcement.

18. To reinforce the mold you need wire cloth, which usually has four square holes per square inch. Cut a strip about 1 inch (25 mm) wide and 8 or 10 inches (20 to 25 cm) long.

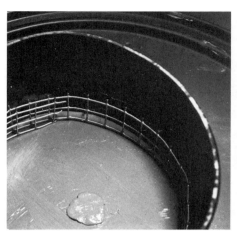

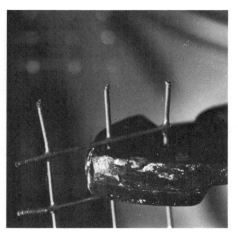

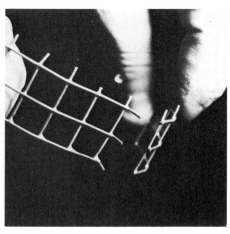

19. Put the rubber circle back on the board. Make a circle out of the wire cloth and place it inside the rubber circle. Fit it in such a way that it stays about ¼ inch (6 mm) away from the rubber wall on all sides. Mark the overlap on the wire circle.

20. Take out the wire strip and with pliers remove one or two of the vertical wires from one end, leaving the horizontal wires projecting.

21. To lock the ends, bend the horizontal wires at this end into a right angle.

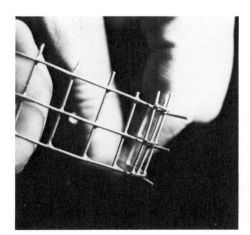

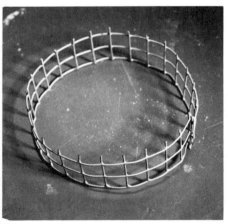

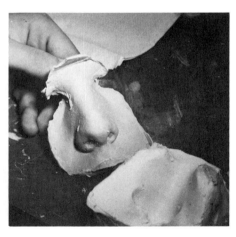

22. Pass them through the holes of the other end, where you marked the overlap, and with pliers bend them flat to lock the ends.

23. Now you have a wire circle.

24. By this time the plaster positive of the nose should be dry. Remove the alginate, and you have a perfect positive of the subject's nose.

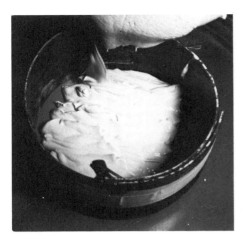

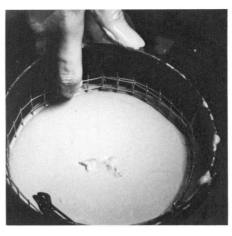

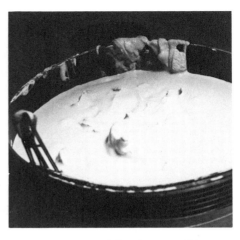

25. Mix a thick batch of plaster and pour it inside the rubber wall to a depth of about 1 inch (25 mm). If the mold is on a movable board, hold the board at the corners and gently shake it to spread the plaster evenly inside the circle.

26. Insert the wire cloth inside the rubber wall and press it into the plaster until it touches the bottom. Then gently lift it about ¼ inch (6 mm) and let it stay there.

27. Pour in the rest of the plaster until it covers the top of the wire circle by about ¼ inch (6 mm). This extra plaster is absolutely necessary; otherwise you will have trouble carving keys in the mold (see steps 31–33).

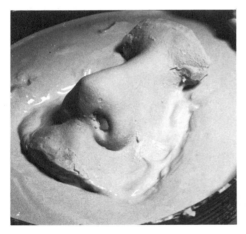

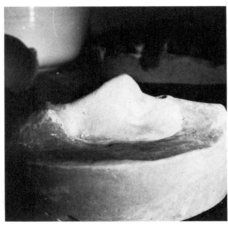

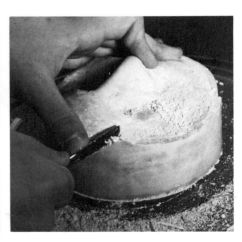

28. If the plaster is very soft, allow it to set a little. Then gently place the positive nose in the center of the circle (nose pointing upward) and press it in to hold it. Do not drown the nose in the plaster; you are simply making a base for it.

29. Remove the rubber wall when the plaster is set but not totally dry. With a spatula add some plaster to the top and bottom ends of the nose and level if off. (This can also be done while the rubber wall is still around the mold.)

30. Use a surgical knife to smooth out the edges and the surface of the mold.

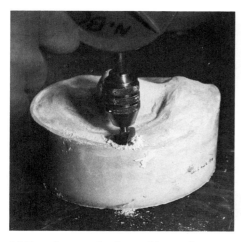

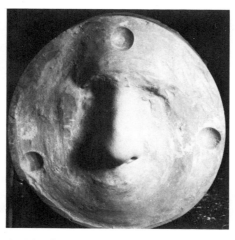

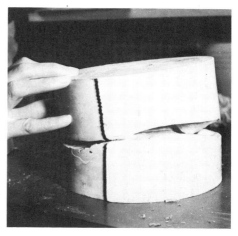

31. In order to make the positive and negative molds fit together exactly, you must make "keys" to lock them together. With a drill and a ¾-inch (19-mm) round router bit, make the keys as close to the edge of the mold and as far away from the cutting edge (see Chapter Six) as you can. If you do not have a router bit, use a knife. (Another kind of key will be explained later in this chapter.)

32. The distance between the keys must be exactly the same.

33. If not, when you have finished the modeling and have cast and placed the positive and the negative together, they may look right. But if you press one side, you see that the top mold rocks up and down.

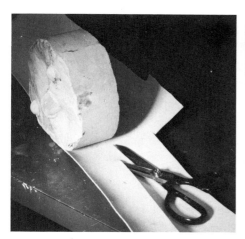

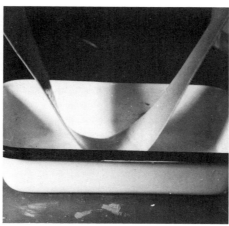

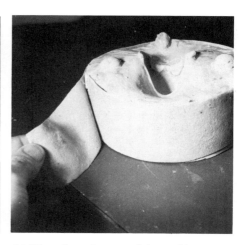

34. To reinforce the mold from the outside for extra protection, cut a strip of Celastic to fit the height of the mold all around. Rub a little petroleum jelly on your fingers before working with Celastic to keep them from getting sticky. Allow at least 2 to 3 inches (5 to 8 cm) at the end for overlap.

35. Soak the strip of Celastic in acetone.

36. Wrap the strip around the mold. Press the overlap to seal it, and let the strip dry. It shrinks as it dries and holds the mold tightly, so that if there are any cracks in the mold it won't fall apart.

The mold is now ready for modeling.

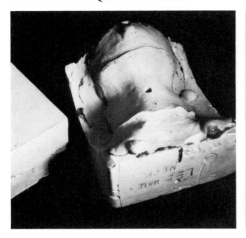

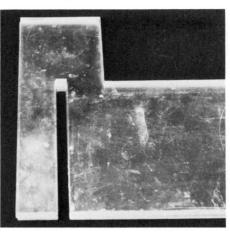

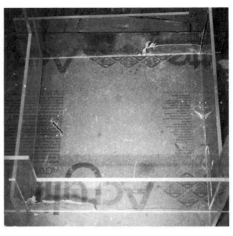

1. Molds may be made square instead of round; the shape of the mold has nothing to do with the way it works.

2. The photograph shows four pieces of ¼-inch (6-mm) acrylic cut 16 inches (40½ cm) long by 8 inches (20½ cm) wide, which can be used to make a square or rectangular mold. (If you use wood instead of acrylic or Plexiglas, you must cover the walls with petroleum jelly before pouring in plaster. But remember that the wetness of the plaster eventually makes wooden pieces useless.) Each piece has a tower-shaped section at one end and a ¼-inch (6-mm) cutout about 5⅛ inches (13 cm) high.

3. When they are locked together, these four pieces can give you all sizes of square molds.

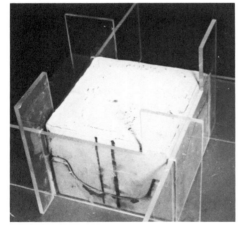

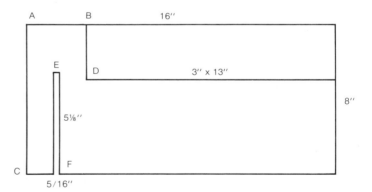

4. They also create rectangular molds. Use masking tape at the joints and some clay where the pieces meet the acrylic board underneath to prevent them from sliding open with the pressure of the plaster inside.

The accompanying diagram is only a guide for making these pieces. You can change the measurements as you wish. Cut a large piece of acrylic to be used as a board under the molds as well. The following instructions are for a sheet of acrylic 16 inches (40½ cm) long and 8 inches (20½ cm) wide.

A. Make a mark (*B*) 3 inches (7½ cm) to the right of the upper left-hand corner (*A*) and another mark 3 inches (7½ cm) down from *B* (*D*).

B. At the bottom center of section *CABD* mark a narrow opening (*EF*) 5⅛ inches (13

cm) long and slightly wider than ¼ inch (6 mm), which is the thickness of the acrylic. Slightly wider, about 5/16 inch (7 mm), is a good width for easy locking of the pieces. Cut out this slot as accurately and as straight as you can.

C. Then cut out and discard the entire 3 by 13 inch (7½ by 33 cm) area or leave it, if you prefer. You will have a piece of acrylic like the ones shown above. Repeat these steps to make the other three sections. For smaller molds cut smaller pieces.

THE SIDES OF THE FACE: MAKING A NEGATIVE

The following technique for casting the sides of the face can also be used for casting the forehead, chin, upper lip, neck, and double chin from the life mask.

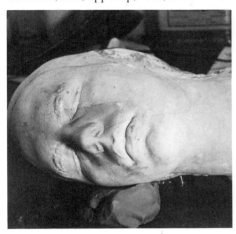

1. Place the life mask on its side and secure it with clay.

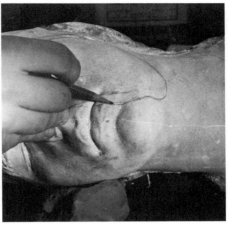

2. Mark 1 inch (25 mm) or so beyond the area of the face needed for the prosthetic piece you have in mind.

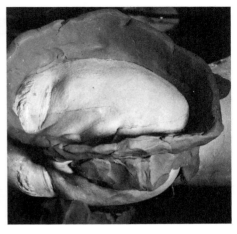

3. Make a clay wall as explained in steps 2–6 on page 26.

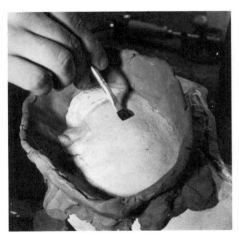

4. Brush petroleum jelly over the area side the clay wall. Make sure there are openings under the clay through which plaster can escape.

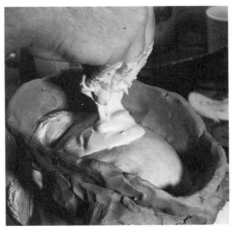

5. Mix a small batch of plaster and make sure there are no lumps or air bubbles trapped in it. (For these negatives you can use Hydrocal instead of B-11 or Ultracal 30.) Then gently pour or brush it inside the clay wall, until you have a layer about ½ inch (13 mm) thick.

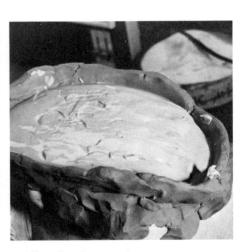

6. Allow the plaster to dry.

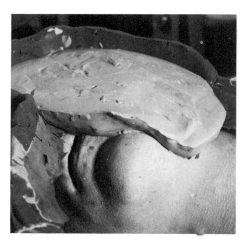

7. When the plaster is totally dry, remove the clay wall.

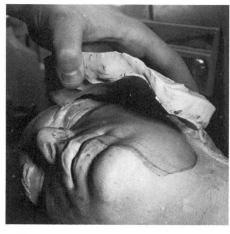

8. Very gently remove the plaster piece. If it is not totally dry, it will break during separation. This technique is also known as a snap mold.

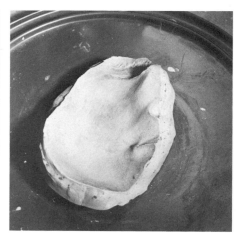

9. What you have now is a negative of the side of the subject's face, taken from the life mask.

THE SIDES OF THE FACE: MAKING A POSITIVE

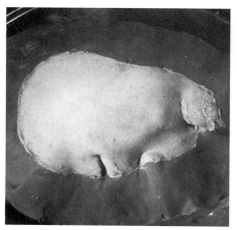

10. Place the negative face up on a board on your worktable. With either water clay or used modeling clay, build an extension around the negative. The extension has to match the shape and height of the plaster piece; one side might be higher than the other. Smooth the clay as best as you can. Make the distance between the edge of the plaster and the outer edge of the clay the same all around, about 1½ inches (4 cm).

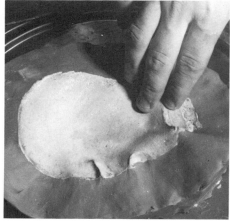

11. When you are satisfied with the shape you have created, rub the entire surface of the plaster and its extension sparingly with petroleum jelly.

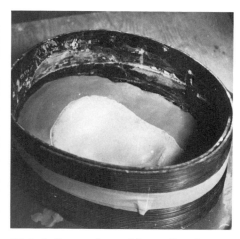

12. As before, make a rubber wall to fit around the negative and secure it with masking tape. Make sure the clay touches the rubber. If the edges do not touch, the plaster will escape.

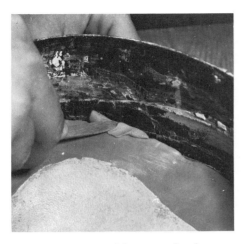

13. If there are gaps, either press the clay with your fingers to touch the wall, or add bits of clay to the open areas and smooth them. If you are using wire reinforcement, prepare it now (see steps 18–23 on pages 28–29).

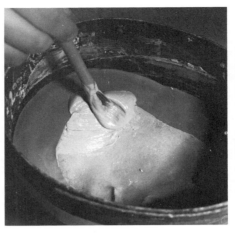

14. Mix a small batch of plaster. (Because this positive mold eventually will be placed in the oven, use either Ultracal 30 or B-11.) Make sure the plaster has no air bubbles or lumps in it; then brush the first layer onto the mold and let it set. Apply the second layer in the same way, rinse the brush in cold water, and mix another batch of plaster.

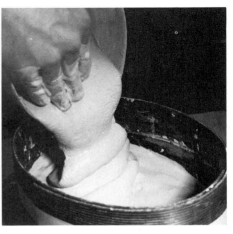

15. Gently pour the plaster in from one side and let it spread by itself over the surface of the mold. Continue this until the plaster is about ½ inch (13 mm) thick.

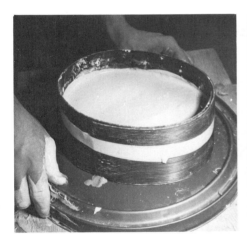

16. Continue adding plaster, with additional batches as needed, until it is no more than 2 inches (5 cm) thick, or until it covers the wire reinforcement by about ¼ inch (6 mm). Then hold the board under the mold and gently rock it back and forth to release any air bubbles trapped under the surface and to make the top of the mold smooth.

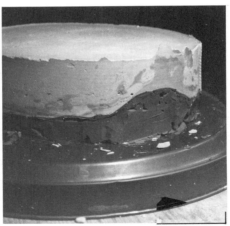

17. After the plaster has gone through its chemical changes—first hot, then cold—remove the rubber wall.

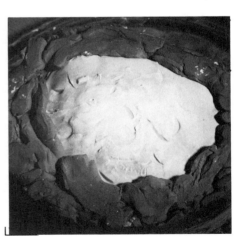

18. Turn the mold upside down.

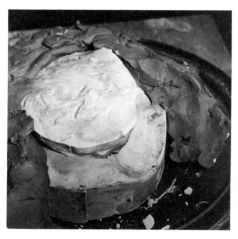

19. Remove the clay.

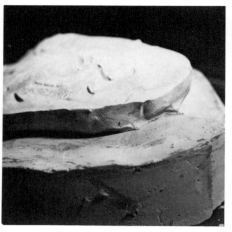

20. Now the positive mold is at the bottom with the negative attached to it. Remove the negative.

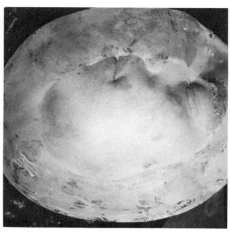

21. The positive of the left side of the subject's face is ready for modeling.

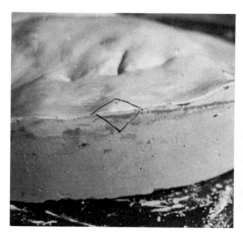

22. Before the plaster dries totally, you must cut the keys. For the nose we used round keys. For this mold we shall use notches. (You can use whichever you prefer on any piece.) Mark a *V* shape about ¾ inch (19 mm) deep on the surface and the side wall of the mold.

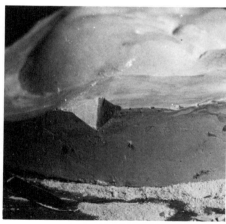

23. Cut through the plaster with a surgical knife or a rasp. The result is a deep notch.

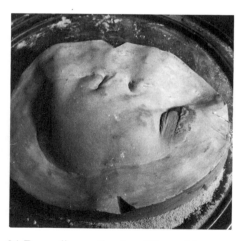

24. Depending on the size of the mold, you can make three or four notches. Make sure that they are equidistant.

The mold is ready for modeling.

There is another way to make these positives that dispenses with a few steps; it will be discussed at the end of Chapter Three. You can use alginate to make the negatives from the life mask, but then you must make a positive and set it in a block. This technique is not advantageous if you have to duplicate a piece more than once for different ages; with a plaster negative you can make as many positives as you wish.

THE THREE-PIECE MOLD

When you need a one-piece prosthetic appliance to cover the sides of the face and the neck, you can make a three-piece mold, or you can use the entire life mask as it is. You can also use three separate pieces covering the sides of the face, the double chin, and neck overlapping. This chapter demonstrates making a three-piece mold.

■■■ MATERIALS AND EQUIPMENT ■■■

Positive of the subject's face

Pencil

Modeling clay or water clay

Spatula

Modeling tools

⅜-inch (9-mm) brushes

Plaster (Ultracal 30 or B-11)

Petroleum jelly

Rubber or plastic bowls

Water

Japanese brush

Surgical knife

Rasp

Burlap

Wooden handle 6 inches (15 cm) long, ½ inch (13 mm) in diameter

Surform tool

Rubber matting

Milk glass or ¼-inch (3-mm) plastic sheet

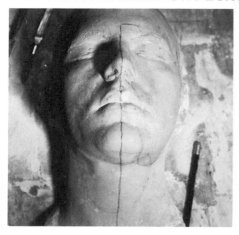

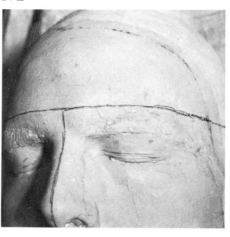

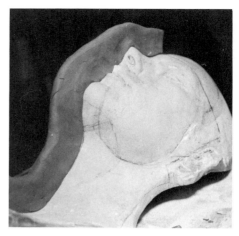

1. Place the subject's life mask, facing up, on a board on your worktable. Draw a straight line down the center from the eyebrows over the nose, upper and lower lips, and chin, ending at the Adam's apple, or below it if necessary.

2. Draw another line straight across the forehead, touching the tip of the first line, passing over the eyebrows, and ending in front of the ears.

3. Make a clay wall about ½ inch (13 cm) wide and 1 inch (25 mm) high, as explained in Chapter Two (steps 2–6, page 26), and place it to the *left* of the center line, not on top of it. Press the clay down to make sure it will not fall. Press lumps of clay behind it for reinforcement. It is very important that this center wall be smooth and, where it touches the mold, clean and straight. There should be no gaps or openings, no matter how small, where the clay touches the life mask.

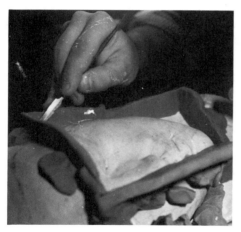

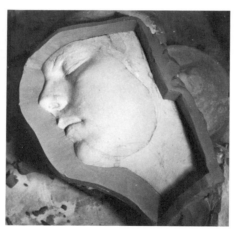

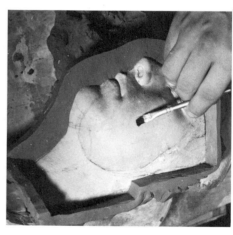

4. When the wall is secure, turn the mold onto its side. Place the side of the face you are not casting on the table and secure it so that it doesn't rock in any direction. Make more clay walls of the same size and place one piece behind the pencil line above the subject's left eyebrow, facing you. Continue this clay wall, passing the subject's left ear, down the neck. Connect it to the center wall at the neckline.

5. It is important, as we have said before, that the edge of the clay wall where it touches the plaster be smooth and clean with no gaps through which the plaster can escape. You should make the seal tight with a modeling tool instead of your fingers. Remember to reinforce all the walls from behind.

6. Brush petroleum jelly sparingly over the entire surface of the plaster inside the clay wall.

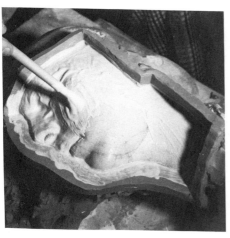

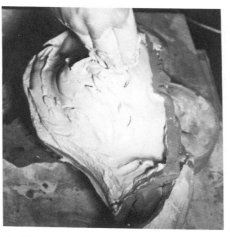

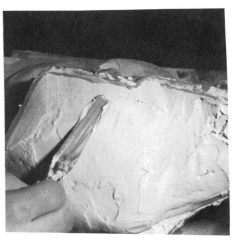

7. Mix a small batch of creamy-smooth plaster, take the air bubbles out of it, and brush it on the mask inside the wall. You may pour it in if you like, but because of the critical center seam, it is better to use a brush for the first couple of layers. After applying each layer, rinse the brush in clear water; then get close to the mold and blow on the wet plaster as hard as you can to break any air bubbles that might be trapped beneath the surface (see step 5, page 21).

8. While the first couple of layers are setting, mix a larger batch of plaster. Make the consistency thick enough that you can gently pour the plaster inside the clay wall. Always pour from one corner and allow the plaster to spread slowly and evenly to prevent trapping air bubbles.

9. Mix more plaster as it is needed, and add it to the previous layer to a thickness of about 1 inch (25 mm). When the plaster is set, smooth the surface with a spatula. Let the plaster dry totally—that is, wait for it to cool.

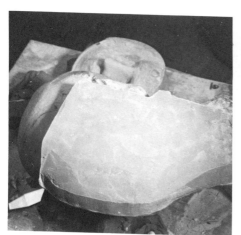

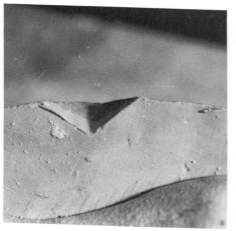

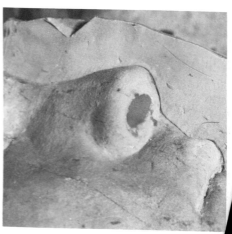

10. Remove the clay wall but not the plaster piece.

11. Turn the mold onto its back, smooth out the top of the center wall, and then, with a surgical knife or wood or plaster rasp, make two notches. Each notch should be about 1 inch (25 mm) wide and ½ inch (13 mm) deep.

12. One notch should be in the area of the nose.

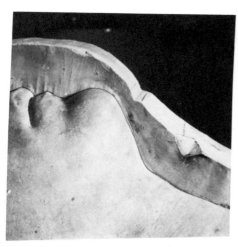

13. The other should be around the neck area.

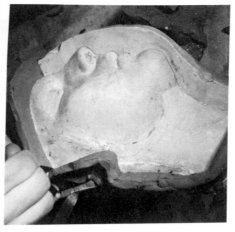

14. Do not remove the mold. Turn the mold to the other side and secure it. Make a clay wall as before, except this time you do not need a clay wall for the center because there is a plaster wall. Place the clay wall behind the line on top of the subject's right eyebrow, extend it all the way down the side of the face and neck, and connect it to the bottom of the plaster wall at the neck-line. Smooth the inside of the clay enclosure, especially where the clay touches the surface of the mold.

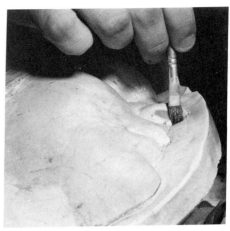

15. With a brush apply petroleum jelly to the entire surface of the mold and the side of the center wall, including the keys, and 1 inch (25 mm) or so beyond.

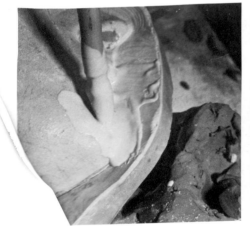

all batch of plaster. As before,
se brush cover the surface of
uple of times. Allow the first
e you apply the second.
batch and do exactly
e other side of the face.
dry totally.

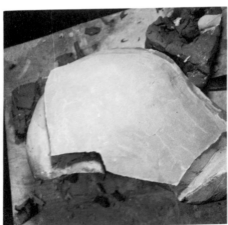

17. Remove all the clay walls.

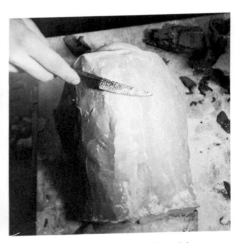

18. Set the mold in its original position. With a file, carefully scrape the plaster at the center seam until the seam is clearly visible.

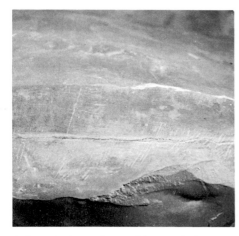

19. Smooth the surfaces of the two halves.

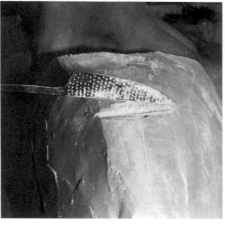

20. With a surgical knife or a wood or plaster rasp (shown), cut two keys at the top of the seam about 2 inches (5 cm) long and ¼ inch (6 mm) deep.

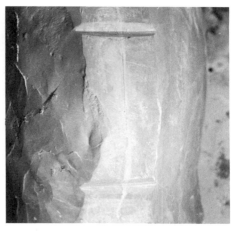

21. Make one at the nose and the other in the neck area, but not on top of or close to the keys you made previously.

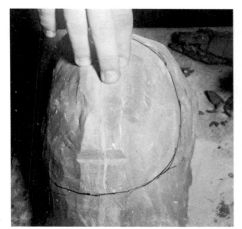

22. Brush off all the plaster dust; then draw a circle over the two sections as shown in the photograph. Include in the circle the two new keys you have just carved over the center seam. Rub petroleum jelly over the entire area inside the pencil mark and 1 inch (25 mm) or so beyond.

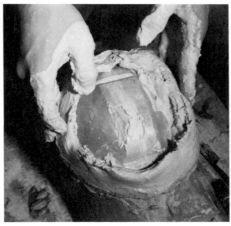

23. Mix a creamy-smooth batch of plaster, saturate a long strip of burlap with it, and place the burlap over the pencil mark in a circle or wall.

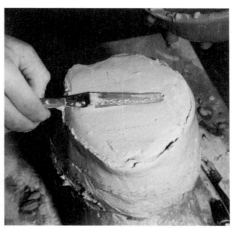

24. When it is set, fill the inside with more plaster to the top of the burlap. Use a spatula to create a flat surface.

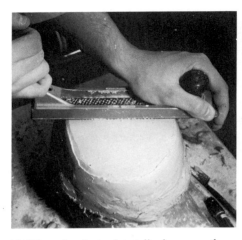

25. When the plaster is totally dry, smooth it out with a rasp, knife, or surform tool.

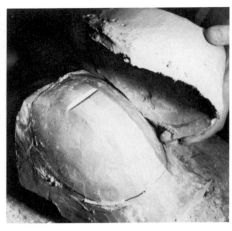

26. Remove the piece you just made and put it aside after it is totally dry.

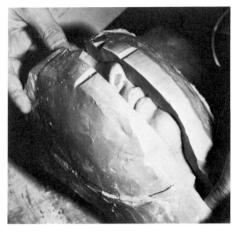

27. Very gently separate the two sections covering the cast of the subject's face. You might need to use a hammer and a surgical knife, but be careful not to break the first set of keys.

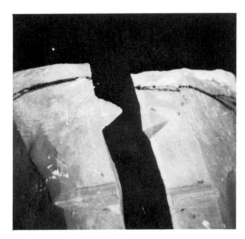

28. First remove the second half of the face you have just cast, the one with the pointed triangles.

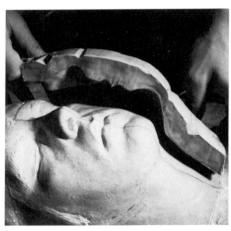

29. Then remove the other half.

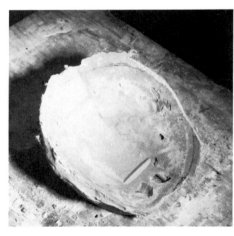

30. Now place the base, the third section, on the table.

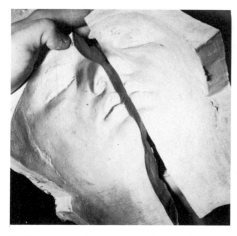

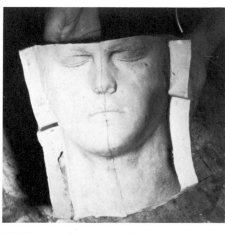

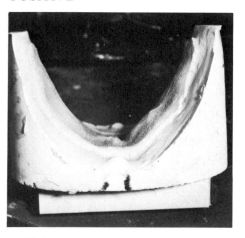

31. Place the other two negatives inside it, first the right side of the face (the one with the pointed triangles), then the other, and make sure the four keys fit tightly.

32. Now you have a negative of the subject's face, from the eyebrows down to the neck, in three pieces. From this you can make as many positive three-quarter life masks as you want.

33. If the positive made from this negative were *U*-shaped, the chances are that when heated it would expand and lose its original shape. This means that the final prosthetic piece would not fit properly.

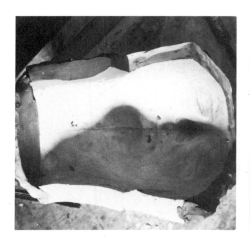

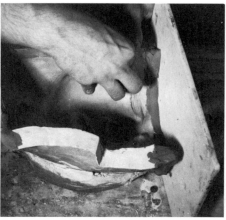

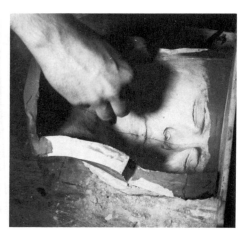

34. To prevent this, close the two ends of the negative with clay walls, wood, acrylic sheet, or milk glass. Here we have built a clay wall at the neck, high enough to be level with the top of the plaster mold.

35. On the other end, which is wider, we used a sheet of milk glass. Both barriers should be erected at right angles to the mold. This means that you must extend the plaster *U* shape to reach the milk glass or the clay wall. Then both have to be reinforced from the back with clay; otherwise the pressure of the plaster would force the walls away from the negative.

36. Apply petroleum jelly to the inside of the mold and to the walls.

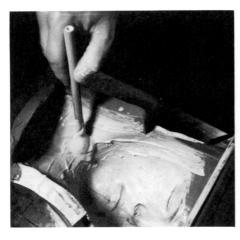

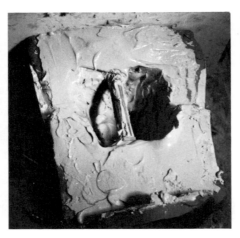

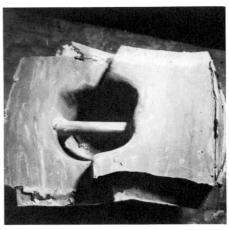

37. Mix a small batch of plaster (Ultracal 30 or B-11) and apply the first couple of layers with a brush. Let it set.

38. Mix a larger batch of plaster and add a little at a time to the mold. When it is about 1 inch (25 mm) thick, add some burlap as reinforcement and cover it with a thick layer of plaster. You must provide a center cavity deep and wide enough for a wooden handle that you can hold to remove the mold (see steps 10–12, page 22).

39. Before the plaster gets totally set, smooth the surface with a spatula or your fingers. Let it dry totally. Remove the walls from both ends.

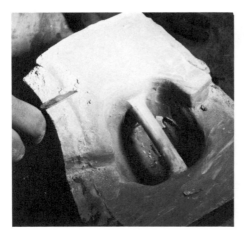

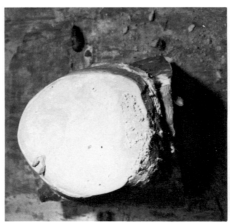

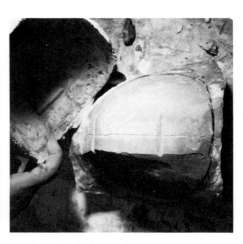

40. Do the last-minute carving and cleaning with a surgical knife or different-size rasps.

41. Turn the mold upside down.

42. Remove the base piece first.

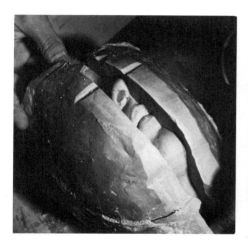

43. Remove the two negatives without breaking the keys.

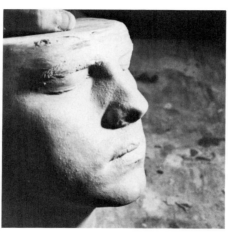

44. Now you have a positive of the subject's face from the forehead to the neck.

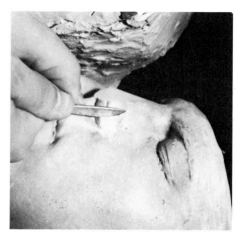

45. At this time you can cut off the subject's nose and make it level with the forehead. You may leave the nose on if you wish to model it in the same mold, but it is not needed. If you know at this time that the outside corners of the nostrils will give you trouble as undercuts (see Chapter Six), use a surgical knife to cut them off, too.

The mold is now ready for modeling.

POSITIVES OF THE NOSE AND CHIN

After making the positive of the subject's face from the three-piece mold, I was asked, "Can't we take the positive of the different parts of the face out of this mold instead of doing what is explained in Chapter Two?" The answer is yes. If you know in advance that in the process of aging you need different parts of the face, it is a good idea to make the three-piece mold first and proceed in the following way.

In this sequence the steps are the same for both the nose and the chin; the photographs show only the chin.

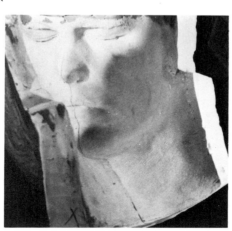

1. Place the three-piece mold on a board on your worktable. Make sure the keys are well in place and there is no separation at the center seam.

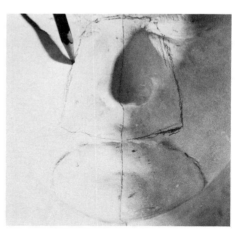

2. Mark about ½ inch (13 mm) beyond the chin (nose) area with pencil.

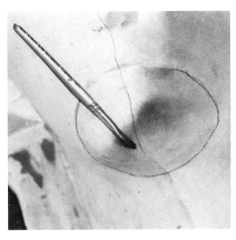

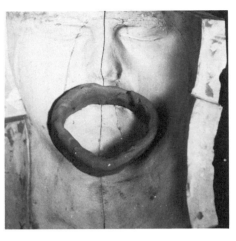

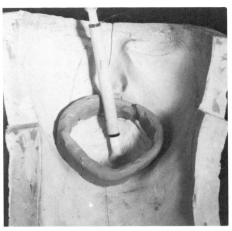

3. Apply petroleum jelly to the area inside the pencil mark without going beyond it.

4. Place a clay wall about 1 inch (25 mm) high around the pencil mark.

5. Mix a small batch of plaster (Ultracal 30) as creamy as you can make it and brush it inside the clay wall. You can gently pour it in, but it is better to brush on the first couple of layers.

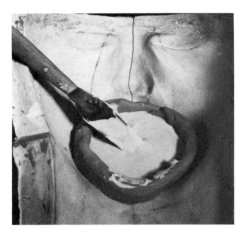

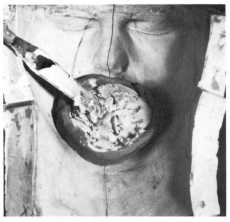

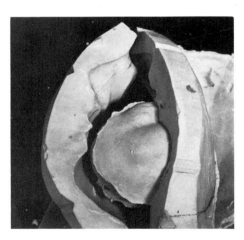

6. While the first layers set, make a larger batch of plaster. Make sure it contains no air bubbles, and then gently pour it into the mold from one side and let it spread to fill the space; or feed the plaster into the mold with a spatula.

7. When the plaster has set, make the surface as uneven as you can.

8. When the plaster is totally dry, gently open the mold and snap out the chin or the nose.

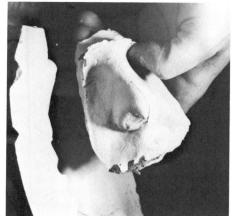

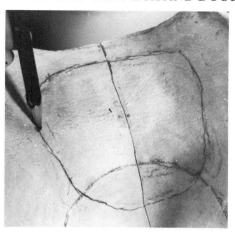

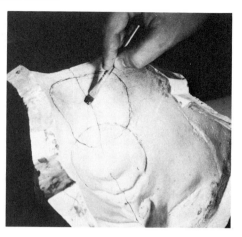

10. For the neck or double chin, put the mold back together and mark the area with pencil.

11. Brush petroleum jelly inside the pencil mark.

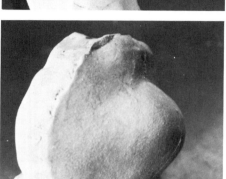

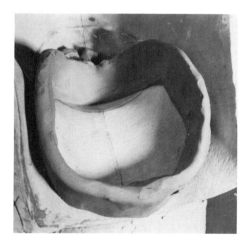

9. What you have now is a positive of the subject's chin or nose.

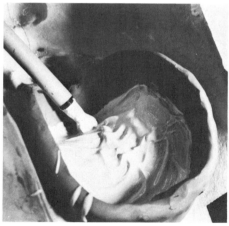

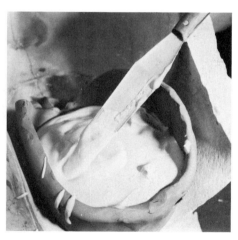

12. Construct a clay wall around the pencil mark.

13. Apply the first couple of layers of plaster with a brush.

14. Add the rest with a spatula or pour it in.

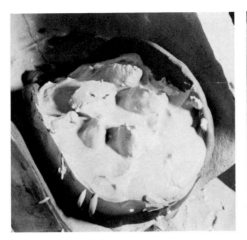 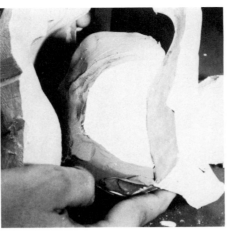 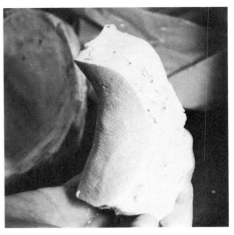

15. When the plaster is set, make the surface uneven.

16. When the plaster is totally dry, open the negative.

17. Snap out the positive of the neck or the double chin.

POSITIVES OF THE SIDES OF THE FACE

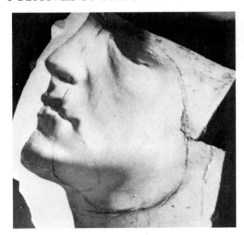 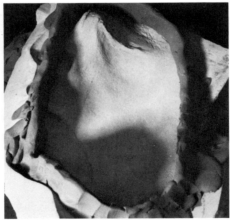 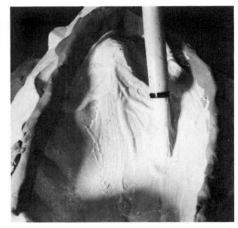

18. For the sides of the face you must separate the halves of the mold. Set the one you are using flat on its back; if necessary, place some used clay under it to keep it level and secure. Mark the area with pencil. (This photograph shows a negative, not a positive, mold.)

19. Place a 1-inch (25-mm) -high clay wall around the pencil mark. Brush petroleum jelly inside the wall.

20. Brush on the first couple of layers of plaster.

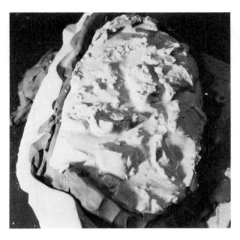

21. When the plaster is set, pour in the rest. When that is set, make the surface uneven.

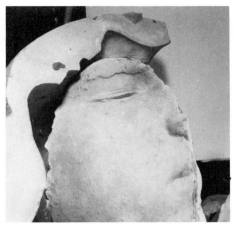

22. When the plaster is totally dry, remove the clay wall and snap out the positive.

To mount these positives in round or square blocks, follow the steps described in steps 16–36, pages 28–31.

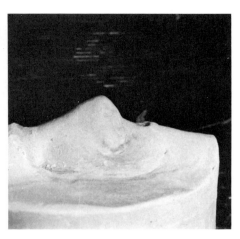

Positive of the nose.

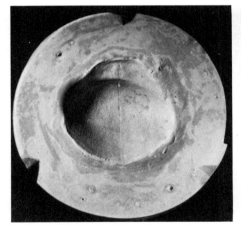

Positive of the chin.

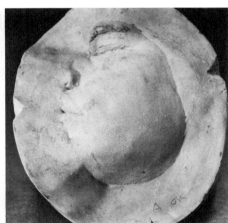

Positive of the side of the face.

Another question must be answered here. Can't the modeling be done over the original life mask before the three-piece mold is made? As we have said, the reason for making a three-piece mold is to create a wraparound foam piece on a smaller or cut-down life mask.

Let's say you have done your modeling over the original mold. If the original life mask is made of Hydrocal, you cannot place it in the oven; therefore, you must first make a positive with Ultracal 30. Then transfer the modeling from Hydrocal mold to it, using either of the techniques explained in Chapter Five.

The next step is to make a negative. If you make it in a three-piece mold, though you don't have to worry about undercuts (see Chapter Six), at the end you will wind up with a seam over the foam piece, unless your modeling is only for the two sides of the face. In fact, it is not a bad idea to use a three-piece mold for the two sides of the face. The seam in the plaster will be in the center, away from the thin edges of the foam. And if you are making a negative without the seam in the center, it's not a three-piece mold. It is either a tub-shaped negative, shown for steps 36 and 39 on page 89, or a *U*-shaped negative, shown for step 33 on page 43, which will soon expand and create thick edges in the foam piece.

CHAPTER FOUR

CASTING HANDS

Because our subject will appear to be very old at the end, it is logical and necessary to age his hands, using the same techniques as for the face, with foam latex. (For intermediate ages, highlight and shadow techniques are best.) Every makeup artist has a favorite technique for casting hands; here is one you can try.

MATERIALS AND EQUIPMENT

Rubber matting

Modeling clay or water clay

Alginate

Petroleum jelly

Rubber or plastic bowls

Rubber spatula

Pitcher of water

Scissors

Surgical knife

Plaster (B-11 or Ultracal 30)

MAKING THE NEGATIVE

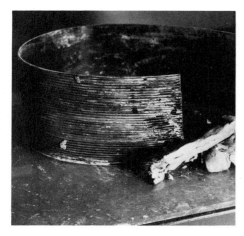

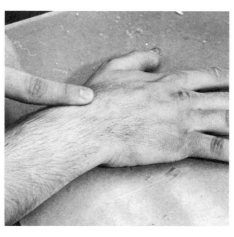

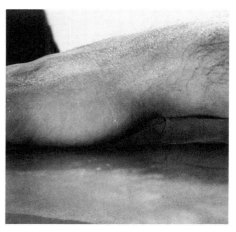

1. Prepare a strip of rubber matting, 24 by 6 inches (61 by 15 cm), to be used as a wall around the hand.

2. If the subject's hands are hairy, apply a coat of petroleum jelly. Place the hand on an acrylic board, making sure that the palm touches the board. The board should be placed at the very edge of your worktable.

3. If you include part of the wrist, as shown here, you will find that directly under the wrist there is a gap. Fill this gap with a piece of modeling clay on both sides and smooth out the edges.

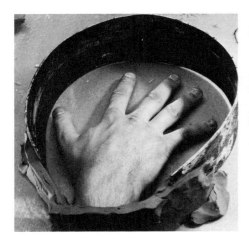

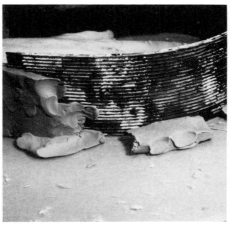

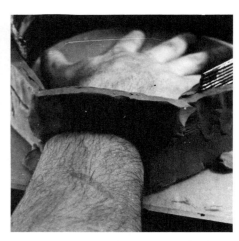

4. Now place the rubber wall around the hand about 1½ inches (4 cm) from the tips of the fingers.

5. Reinforce the wall from the back with some used clay.

6. Add clay to the subject's wrist on both sides and on the top to cut off the flow of the liquid alginate.

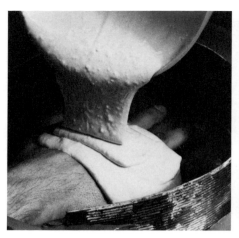 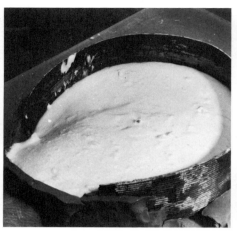 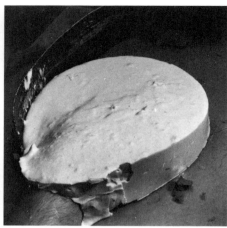

7. Measure and mix the alginate in water at about 70° F. (21° C.). Beat it as fast as you can to a smooth, creamy consistency, so that it is easy to pour. For this you need more water, added right after the first 30 seconds of beating. When the alginate is ready, pour it directly onto the back of the subject's hand and let it spread evenly and slowly all over. Fill the enclosed area to ¼ inch (6 mm) above the highest section of the hand, in this case the wrist. Needless to say, the amount of material you use varies, depending on the size of the hands.

8. Let the alginate set. It is thick, so you probably do not need any plaster backing; however, use your own judgment, and add it if necessary—that is, if the alginate at the wrist area is thin.

9. Remove the rubber wall, but keep it handy.

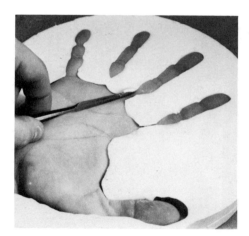 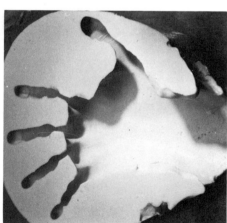

10. Turn over the subject's hand, still in the alginate. If the alginate has gotten under the fingers and the palm of the hand in some areas, cut the excess off with scissors.

11. Gently remove the subject's hand from the alginate, and you have a negative of it.

MAKING THE POSITIVE

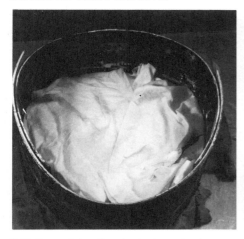

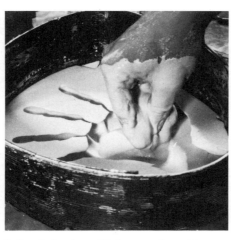

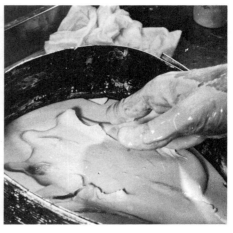

1. Before mixing the plaster to make the positive, place the negative on the board and cover it with wet paper towels.
Put the rubber wall back around the negative and press it to take the same shape. Reinforce it from the back with clay, or use masking tape all around. Mix a batch of plaster smooth and creamy enough to pour easily. Hit the bowl on the table a few times to get rid of air bubbles. Remove the wet towels from the negative and blot up any remaining water with tissues.

2. Gently begin to fill the negative with plaster at the wrist area.

3. Let it float in by itself, and/or aid it to fill the negative by tapping with your fingers.

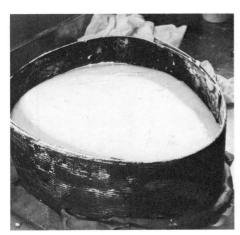

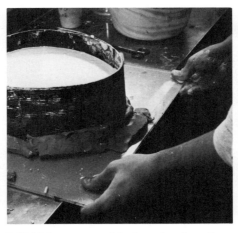

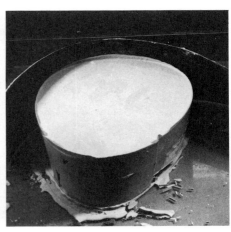

4. Fill the mold to a thickness of at least 1 inch (25 mm) above the surface of the alginate.

5. Hold the corners of the board and gently move it back and forth to level the plaster and raise the air bubbles to the surface.

6. When the plaster has gone through its hot and cold chemical changes and is totally dry, remove the rubber wall.

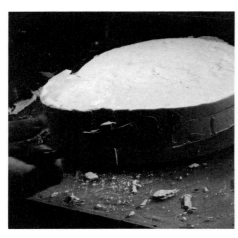

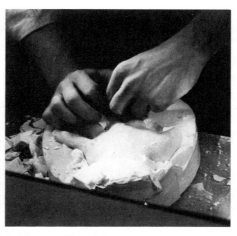

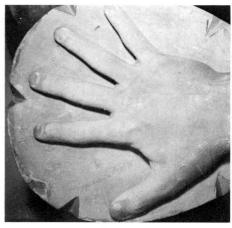

7. Lift the entire mold from the board and turn it upside down.

8. Remove the alginate.

9. Now you have a positive of the subject's hand. Carve keys with a hand drill and ¾-inch (19-mm) router bit, or cut notches with a surgical knife. For this size mold four keys are necessary.

The mold is now ready for modeling. Don't forget the other hand!

ALTERNATE PROCEDURE

Here is another approach to making old-age hands. It is comparatively easier, and its advantages are that you don't cast the subject's hands, you don't have to worry about undercuts (see Chapter Six), and when the foam is made few repairs are needed.

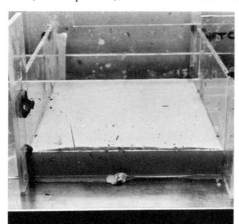

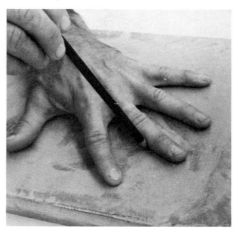

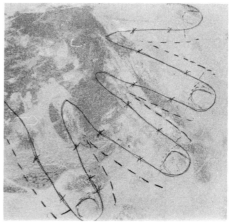

1. Make a plate of Ultracal 30 about 12 by 9½ by 1½ inches (30 by 24 by 4 cm).

2. Place the subject's hand, including part of the wrist, over the plate and mark the fingers, hand, and wrist all around. Keep the fingers as far apart as you can.

3. Now extend the line for each finger from both sides by about ½ inch (13 mm). Mark the new size. You can either include the fingernails in your modeling or use the subject's own fingernails. It is absolutely essential to include them if the foam pieces are going to be glued over surgical gloves and used over and over again, as in the theater.

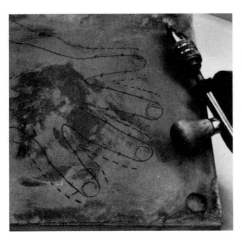

4. Drill four keys.

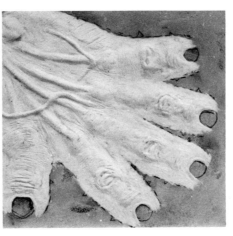

5. Begin the modeling inside this extended area. As in all other modeling, keep the outer edges thin and make sure the modeling is not too thick or so thin that the foam becomes transparent or tears.

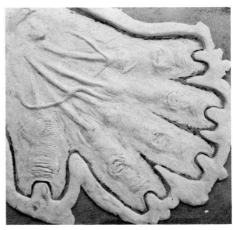

6. When the modeling is finished, create the cutting edge (see Chapter Six).

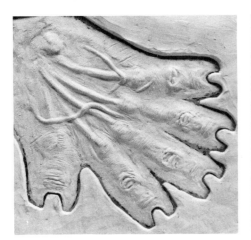

7. Make the overflow (see Chapter Six).

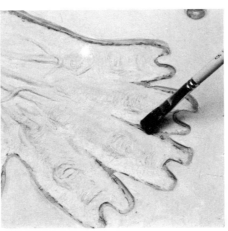

8. Apply cap material or sealer over the clay.

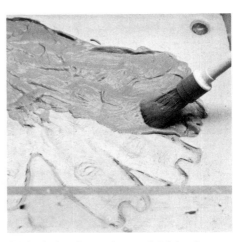

9. Block the plate as in step 1. Make the same amount of plaster as before. Apply the first couple of layers with a brush.

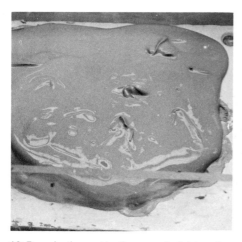

10. Pour in the rest to the same height as the mold and let it dry.

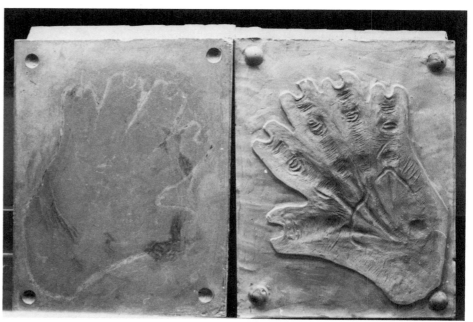

11. When dry, open the two plates. Clean the clay. You now have a positive and a negative, ready for foam.

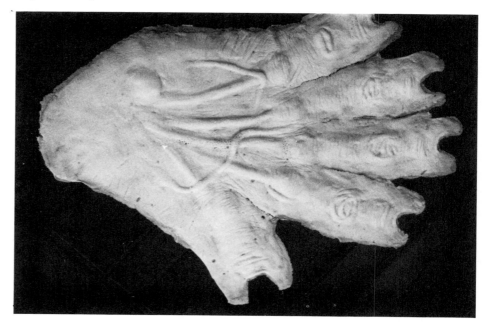

12. Here is the modeled hand in foam. (The process of making foam is fully discussed in Chapter Nine, and application and coloring of foam are described in Chapter Ten.)

PART TWO:
MODELING

CHAPTER FIVE
MODELING AND MODELING TOOLS

There are two basic approaches to modeling in the field of makeup. One is the "look-alike" type—that is, the subject is made up to look like someone else: Abraham Lincoln, Queen Anne, Albert Einstein, or some other famous person. A tremendous amount of research is required for this. In most cases the makeup artist has to search for paintings or photographs that show the person full face and in profile in a particular period and at a certain age. Working from the selected pictures, the makeup artist must model the likeness of the person over the subject's life mask. This requires trained eyes and hands and, needless to say, knowledge of sculpture.

The other approach is "freehand modeling," in which the makeup artist is asked to make the subject older or younger. This approach is much easier because a likeness is not required; nevertheless, it requires the same amount of accuracy and attention to detail. In this case the makeup artist works either from memory or from photographs of old faces. It is best to follow the subject's muscle and bone structure, visualizing what would happen to his face at different ages.

If you are modeling a look-alike mask and your subject's face is smaller than that of the character, you must create the look, not by making your subject's face oversized, but by scaling down the character's features to fit the subject's physical build. When you are working from photographs, do not model a face with an expression on it, such as laughter or anger. Model the face in a relaxed, natural manner; let the actor create the expressions.

In this book we shall not discuss the modeling itself; it is taken for granted that you know how to sculpt. This chapter describes the tools that are useful to the makeup artist.

MODELING TOOLS

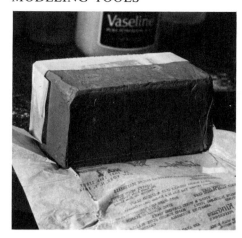

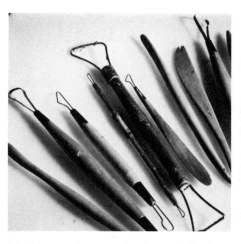

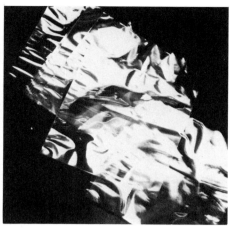

You need Roma Plastilina clay for modeling. It comes in white or gray green. You can purchase each color in soft no. 1, medium no. 2, medium firm no. 3, and very hard no. 4. Some makeup artists prefer to use white clay. Because it is used over a white mold, the finished product looks much more natural than the startling difference of dark modeling clay over a white mold. Some makeup artists like soft clay; others, medium or hard. The kind you use is up to you. No matter which type you choose, however, use it all the way through the piece you are working on. If you mix types, smoothing out the surface becomes much harder.

Modeling tools are made of wood, plastic, or wire. Any art-supply store or sculpture house has available what you need. There is no particular type of tool for a particular part of the face; you must experiment to find the best one for a specific area. When you have become more experienced, you'll select one or two favorites that can do everything you want.

Pieces of cellophane paper are excellent for texturing clay models.

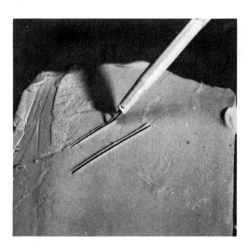

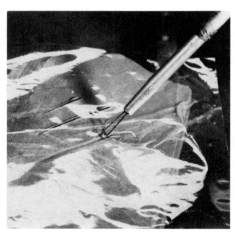

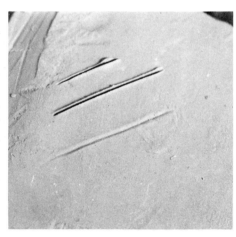

There are times that in the absence of proper texturing materials you have to use sharply pointed tools. When you scratch clay with one of these, you get a deep cut with sharp edges; it is difficult to soften such lines to look like real skin texture.

Instead, place a piece of cellophane paper between the clay and the modeling tool.

The cut or wrinkle made this way has soft edges.

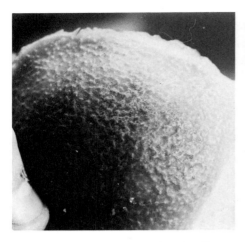

Orange peel is good for creating the effect of porous skin.

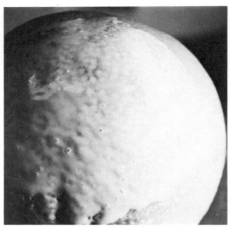

To make one, select an orange or grapefruit with good, porous peel. Cover a section that you like most with ten or fifteen layers of liquid latex. Dry each layer separately.

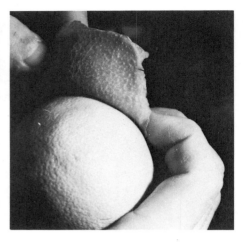

When the latex is totally dry, peel it off.

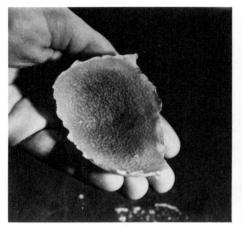

Turn it inside out.

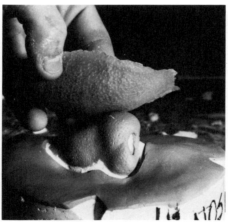

To use it, place it over the clay model and press.

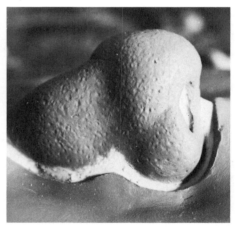

The pressure you use depends on how hard or soft the clay is and how deep you want the pores to be.

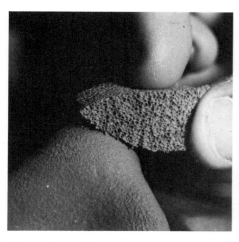

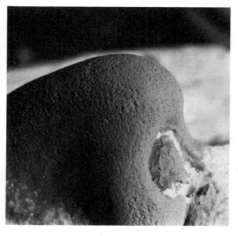

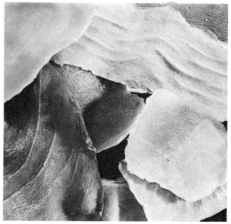

Pieces of red rubber sponge can be used like orange skin. Place a piece over the clay and press.

The result is a much softer porous skin than the orange peel produces. Which one is better I cannot tell you; the choice depends on the character you are creating and the kind of skin needed. You must also consider whether a more subtle effect will wash out in the lighting to be used.

The pieces in this photograph are made of latex, so we shall call them latex stamps. They are impressions of real wrinkles on the forehead, lines on the neck or face, goose pimples on the neck, and fine skin textures of real people. They were not modeled by a makeup artist; they were taken from people's faces or life masks. They are used to give clay models a natural texture and look. To make your own, find people with skin textures and/or wrinkles that you like, and ask if you may cast those parts of their faces. This is the only way to build a stock of latex stamps.

MAKING A LATEX STAMP

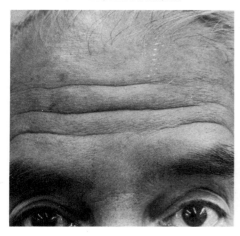

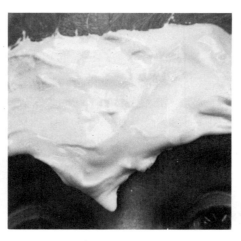

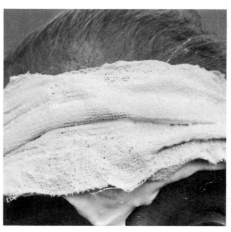

As an example, we shall demonstrate how to make a latex stamp of this man's forehead.

1. Seat the subject in a makeup chair with an adjustable headrest. Rub petroleum jelly on his eyebrows, eyelashes, and hairline. If he has long hair, tape or pin it back. Mix 70 grams of alginate with 200 ml of warm water and apply the mixture to the subject's forehead. The thicker you make it, the faster it will set, and the chances of its running down his face are less.

2. When the alginate is set, cover it with a few layers of plaster bandage. Press each layer to take the shape of the alginate.

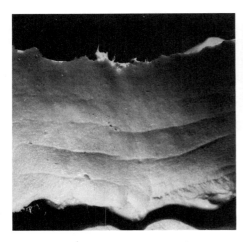

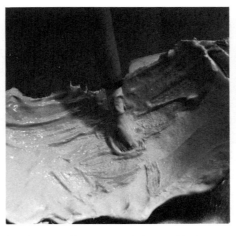

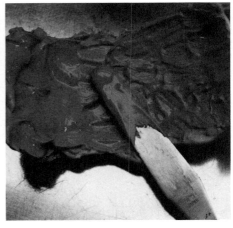

3. When the plaster bandages are dry, remove the entire piece. If the subject did not move his forehead while the alginate was wet, you will have obtained the exact impression of his forehead.

4. Mix a small amount of plaster (Hydrocal) and brush a couple of layers inside the alginate. Let each layer set, but not dry, before the next. (Rinse the brush after each use.)

5. Now mix another small batch of plaster. With a spatula go over the first couple of layers and build a ½-inch (13-mm) thickness all over. Let it dry totally.

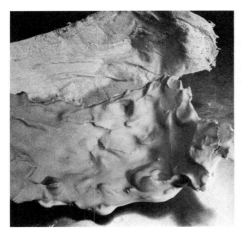

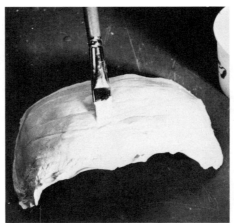

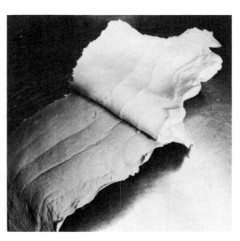

6. Remove the plaster bandages and the alginate; you will have a positive of the man's forehead.

7. To make a latex stamp of it, apply at least ten to fifteen layers of liquid latex over the plaster positive. Let each layer dry before you apply the next. To protect your brush, before each use wet it, rub it over a cake of soap, press it on a paper towel to get rid of excess water, and then dip it into the latex. While the latex dries, rinse the brush in clean water.

8. When the latex is dry, peel it off the plaster. The result is a latex stamp of the forehead in negative form.

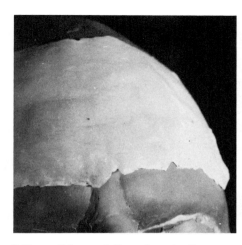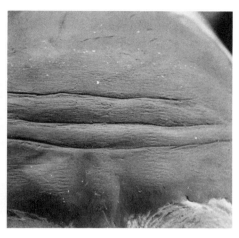

9. To use it for modeling, place the latex stamp over the smooth clay forehead and press.

10. You will get the exact impression of the man's forehead on the clay. It might need touching up here and there, but it looks very natural. The same technique can be used for any part of the face and neck.

CHAPTER SIX

UNDERCUTS, CUTTING EDGE, AND OVERFLOW

When you bite into an apple, your teeth create what is known as an undercut. The only way you can separate the portion of the fruit that is inside your mouth from the rest of the apple is by breaking off the section held by your teeth. That is exactly what happens to a two-piece mold. When one side accidentally gets hold of a part of the other side and won't let go, one or the other will break when the pieces are separated by force. This chapter is about undercuts in mold making and how to avoid them.

UNDERCUTS

Let's say you have finished modeling a nose, and you have cast it to get the negative. When you try to separate the positive and the negative, however, they do not open.

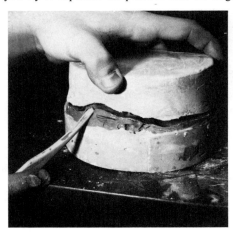

1. You use force to open the molds.

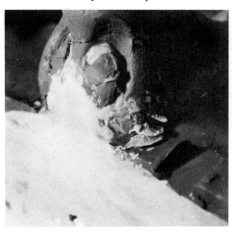

2. You wind up with a damaged negative or positive that cannot be used. You must begin the modeling all over, this time watching out for *undercuts*.

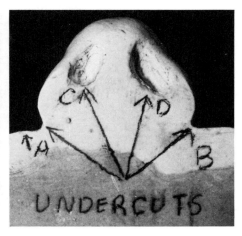

3. This photograph shows a cross section of the mold of a nose. There are four areas of undercuts, at each outer corner of the nostrils (*A* and *B*) and the two nostrils themselves (*C* and *D*).

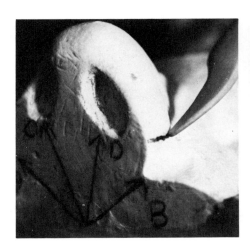

4. The undercuts at the corners (*A* and *B*) start at the middle of the curve of the nostril, where it begins to turn under, and go to the very corner. The nostrils (*C* and *D*) in this mold are undercuts because they are too deep-set, about ⅛ inch (3 mm).

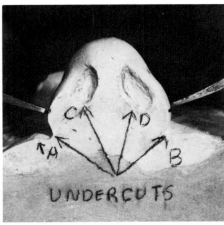

5. To demonstrate why undercuts cause trouble, we place calipers at the beginning of the curve of the nose and pull upward.

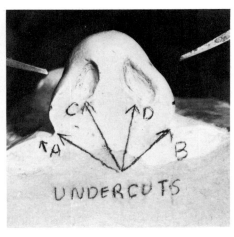

6. The mold stays where it is, but the calipers move.

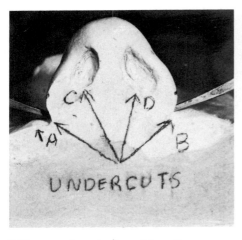

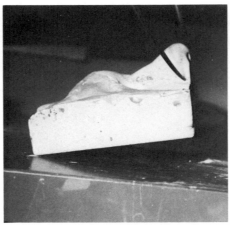

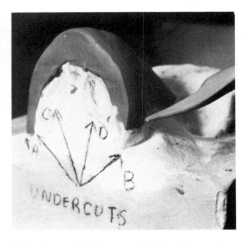

7. Now we place the tips of the calipers at the corners of the nose, hold tight, and lift.

8. We lift the nose as well. The calipers are locked in the corners below the curve, where the undercuts are. Plaster poured over the nose gets below the same curves at the corners, so that the two molds lock together and will not open unless one side or the other breaks.

9. Let's see what happens during the modeling of the nose. Finish modeling at the center of the curve, as shown.

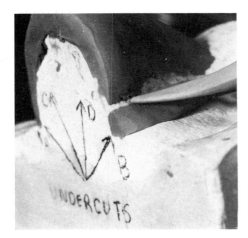

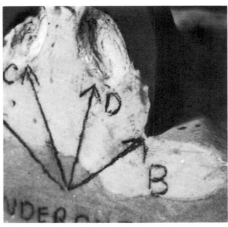

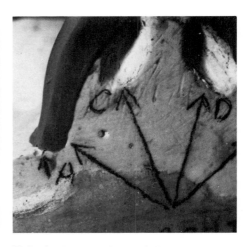

10. You must create the cutting edge (see pages 69–70) as close to the modeled area as possible, and even then you must make sure that it does not fall where the nose begins to curve under.

11. Even if you pass the curve and bring the modeling all the way down to the corners, as shown in the *B* corner, the undercut still exists.

12. In the *A* corner the modeling is thicker, thus filling the corners and preventing breakage. We shall finish modeling this nose and then cast it. In most cases, the modeling does not have to be thick.

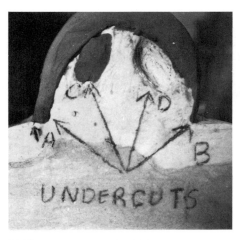

13. Here you can see the difference between the two sides. We have even filled one nostril.

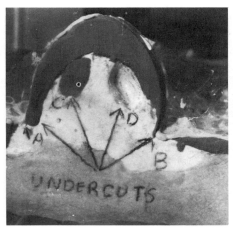

14. Here the mold is shown behind a clear acrylic wall so that you can see exactly what happens. After the plaster is brushed and poured inside the frame and over the modeling, on the *A* side the plaster stays away from the corner, whereas it goes all the way into the *B* corner, like the tip of the calipers. (Under normal circumstances the plaster would fill the open nostril as well, but here because of the cutaway this does not happen.)

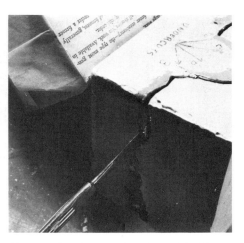

15. After the plaster is dry, the mold will not open and must be forced.

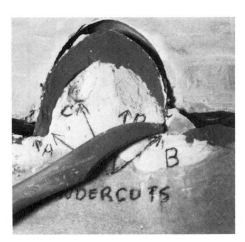

16. As you can see, the *B* corner is chipped; the modeling must be done over. This time we know better.

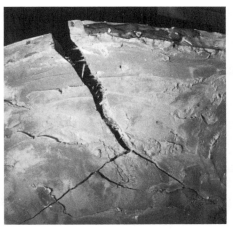

17. A mold like this one must be discarded because of the carelessness of the mold maker. It is absolutely necessary to be aware of where the undercuts are in each face.

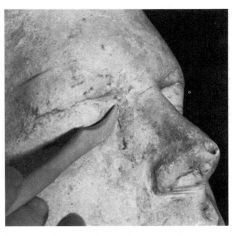

18. In addition to the undercuts at the nostrils and the corners of the nose, we find them at the corners of the eyes, under the eyebrows, . . .

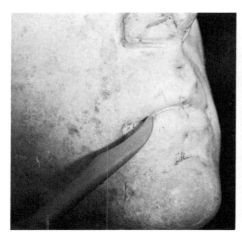

19. . . . between the lips, . . .

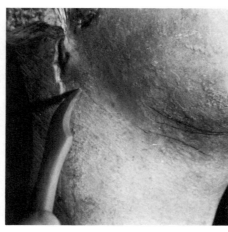

20. . . . under and near the ears, where the jawbones are, . . .

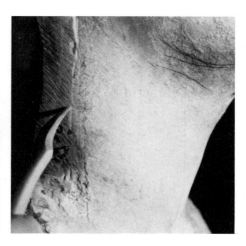

21. . . . at the neck where it begins to curve back, . . .

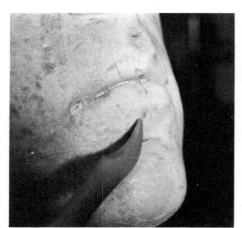

22. . . . under the lower lip, . . .

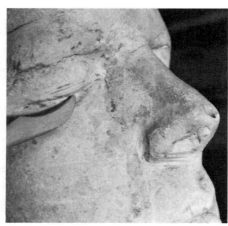

23. . . . and under the lashes in closed eyes.

In each face the undercuts are in different places. You must take care of them before or during the modeling. Some undercuts, such as those shown in photos 18, 19, 22, and 23, may not cause problems, depending on your modeling and the way you open the molds.

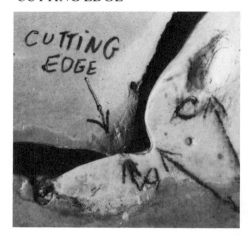

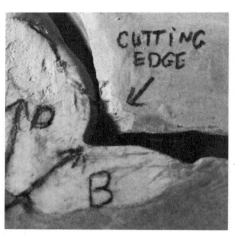

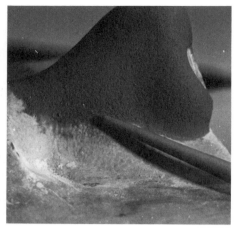

1. Notice in the photograph where the top mold and bottom mold meet next to the corner of the nose; this is called the cutting edge. When you pour foam latex inside the negative mold and place the positive on top, the excess foam is pushed out as you press down. The cutting edge is what stops the flow of the foam and keeps the remaining foam inside the mold—no more and no less than the amount of clay you used to model the piece.

2. On the *B* side of the same mold the upper and lower molds do not meet, so there is nothing to stop the flow of the foam. The result would be a piece of foam with very thick edges—totally unusable.

3. To create the cutting edge you must finish the modeling, texture the piece, and make sure that the edges, where the modeling ends, are as thin as you can make them.

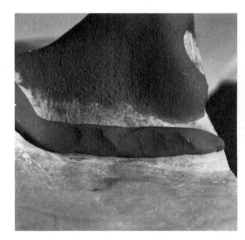

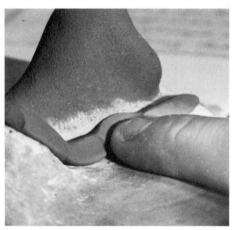

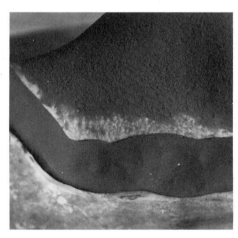

4. Roll a small piece of clean clay on the table to the thickness of a pencil. Place this about ¼ inch (6 mm) away from the edge of the modeled piece all around.

5. With your fingertip press the clay down to adhere to the mold, and at the same time push it about ⅛ inch (3 mm) closer to the edge of the clay model.

6. When you have finished, you will have an exposed area of plaster immediately around the modeled piece. This area does not have to be a straight line; you can make it uneven if you like.

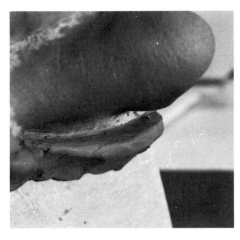

7. The wrong way to build a cutting edge is to make the clay too high, . . .

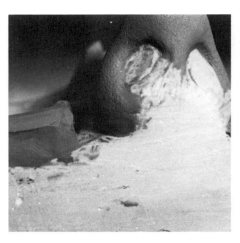

8. . . . or to place it too far away from the edge of the modeled piece.

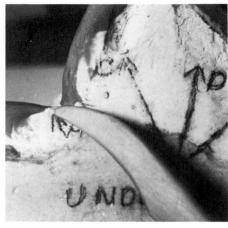

9. Keep it close and shallow to allow the extra foam to escape easily and quickly.

OVERFLOW

When the cutting edge is properly set, you must begin to build the overflow, which is the continuation of the clay you have just placed around the nose for the cutting edge.

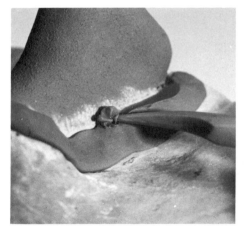

10. To achieve this, cut the excess clay with a modeling tool, and at the same time create the shallowness and close any gaps that might be under the clay at the very edge.

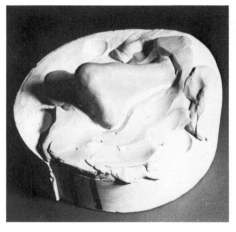

1. Add more clay over the exposed plaster, and with your fingers or tools smooth it as best you can.

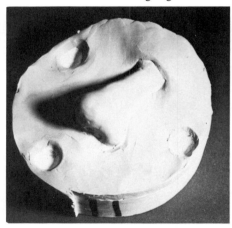

2. Leave the keys exposed like the exposed areas around the nose (cutting edge).

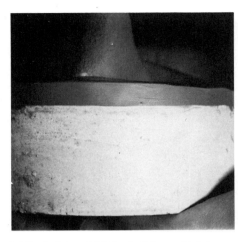 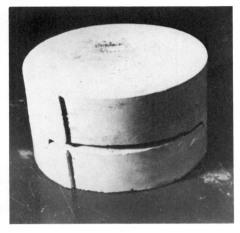

3. The height of this bed of clay, which is known as the *overflow*, should be no less and no more than ¼ inch (6 mm) all around.

4. Why do we call this the overflow? After the modeled piece is cast, and after the clay is removed, there will be a ¼-inch (6-mm) separation between the upper and lower molds. The only areas where the two molds touch are at the keys and the cutting edge. This space makes it easy for the excess foam latex inside the mold to flow away. Hence the term *overflow*.

CHAPTER SEVEN
MODELING AND CASTING SMALL PIECES

Modeling the small pieces should not present any technical difficulties to the experienced makeup artist. There are times, however, when the modeled pieces lose their relationship to the entire face. For instance, a modeled nose may look good by itself over a small round block of plaster, but after the clay nose has been made in foam latex and applied to the subject's face, it might appear out of proportion. Too few makeup artists follow the technique explained here, which prevents this.

In this chapter we show the casting of each piece after the modeling is done. If you are preparing only one or two unrelated pieces, such as a nose and a chin, you can cast them after the modeling is finished, but if you are planning a gradual aging process like the one demonstrated in this book, be aware that the pieces made to portray each age must relate to those made for other ages; certain characteristics must be carried through from one age to the other. It is better to finish all the modeling, and then make sure the relationship between the age and muscle structure is correct before casting the pieces.

MATERIALS AND EQUIPMENT

Pencil

Plastic wrap

Petroleum jelly

Modeling clay

Modeling tools

Spatula

¾-inch (19-mm) brushes

Sealer or cap material

Acetone

Alcohol

Plastic bowls, large and small

Masking tape

Japanese brush

Plaster (B-11 or Ultracal 30)

Surgical knife

Texturing materials (red rubber sponge, orange peel, etc.)

Wire cloth

¾-inch (19-mm) router drill bit and ¼-inch (6-mm) regular drill bit

Electric or hand drill

Wire cutters

Pliers

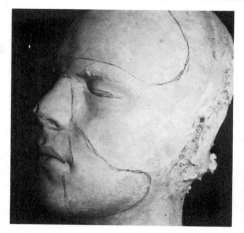

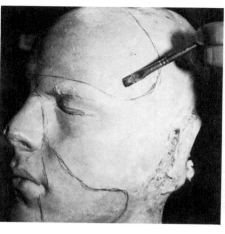

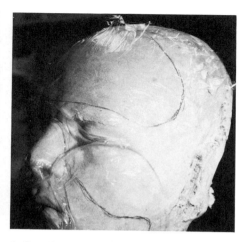

1. Place the subject's life mask on a modeling stand or on your worktable. Mark all the areas of the face for which you are going to make prosthetic pieces. We have marked the forehead, nose, chin, and the sides of the face.

2. Apply a thin coat of petroleum jelly over the marked areas only.

3. Cut pieces of plastic wrap larger than the marked areas and press each one smoothly over the life mask; let them overlap if the areas are close together.

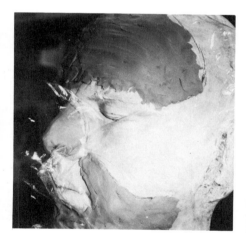

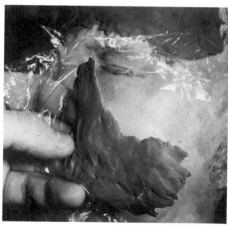

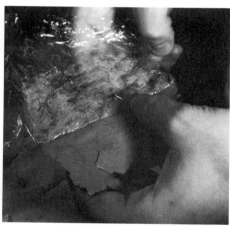

4. Now begin modeling over the plastic wrap. (Be careful when you press the modeling clay over the plastic wrap—it tends to slide around.) This modeling is only to create an overall shape and thickness, not a finished product. You are establishing the correct relationship between the pieces. Needless to say, you must visualize all this with the kind of hair the subject has or that the character is going to wear. If possible, get a similar wig and place it on the life mask.

5. After the rough modeling is finished, very gently lift each piece of plastic wrap.

6. Separate it from the clay. Do not be disturbed if the modeled pieces lose their shape. When they have been placed over their positives, they will return to their intended shape. It is a good idea, however, to paint a coat of cap material or sealer over the clay model before removal to keep the clay together, especially the thin areas.

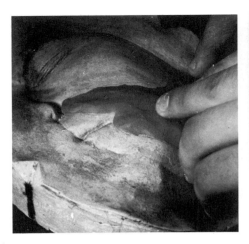

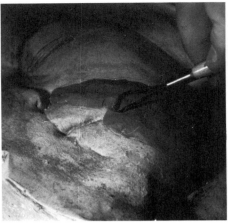

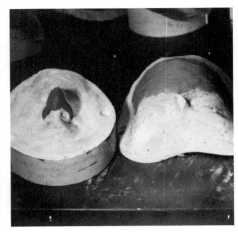

7. Now, coat each positive with petroleum jelly and wipe off most of it. Place the crude modeled pieces over the plaster positives of the same pieces. Press hard to adhere the clay to the plaster.

8. Continue the process of modeling and shaping each area of the clay with your fingers and modeling tools, according to the concept you have in mind for the character. After the clay is secure over the positive and you have made it the right shape, dip a regular stiff bristle brush, cut very short, in alcohol and brush over and around the clay model. This makes the surface much smoother. Then add textures.

9. The same technique applies to the nose, forehead, chin, and neck.

Here is another technique suggested by makeup artist Dick Smith:

Use a clean, fresh, damp life mask of White Hydrocal or dental stone, not Ultrocal 30. Brush on two coats of Al-Cote dental separator or similar alginate-type separator. The surface should feel damp and slick.

Dry the surface with a hair dryer until Plastilina will stick to it. (Sculpture House Roma Plastilina No. 2 is good.) Sculpt the appliance models. Finish details and edges. It helps to paint a layer of plastic cap material over the sculpture except at the very edges.

Submerge the life mask in cold water for about 1 hour. The water reactivates the Al-Cote.

Sometimes the Plastilina loosens when the life mask is shaken under water, but usually you must slide a thin piece of flexible plastic under an edge to pry it off gently. Large areas, such as the forehead, should be cut in half first.

The Plastilina models can be put aside while positives are made of the appropriate area for each model.

Coat each positive with petroleum jelly, wipe off most of it, place the Plastilina model in position, press gently, and smooth down the edges.

Finish repairs, edges, and textures of the model. Make keys and the Plastilina flashing (overflow). Pour up the negatives.

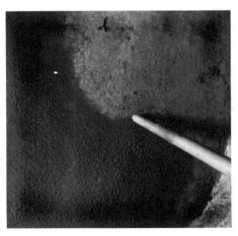

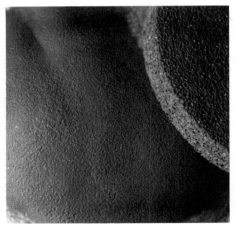

10. It is very important that the edges of the modeling be as thin as you can make them. These thin areas create thin edges on the foam latex, which help camouflage the transition from the piece to natural skin when the appliance is glued to the subject's face. The texture of your modeled pieces must of course match that of the subject's own skin.

11. Select the proper rubber or latex stamp or tools to create the right skin texture. If you find that the pressure of the texturing materials lifts the thin edges of the clay, find a wooden modeling tool with a sharp point, or a pencil, and gently tap the clay at the thin places to give it some skinlike texture. Be sure not to create little holes.

I have been asked how much of this careful texturing will actually be seen. The answer is very little, unless the camera comes close for a head shot. If for no other reason, however, be careful for the sake of the subject: he will feel better if he looks totally natural. Since the effect will wash out in the lighting, it is not a bad idea to exaggerate the textures.

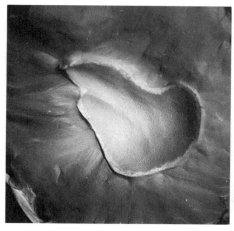

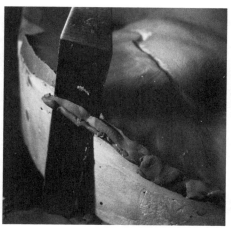

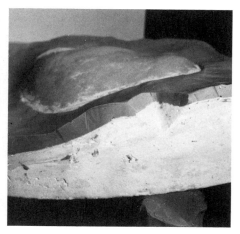

12. After the modeling is finished and the cutting edge is created, extend the overflow areas slightly beyond the edge of the mold.

13. With a metal spatula trim off the excess clay.

14. The result is a smooth and clean mold.

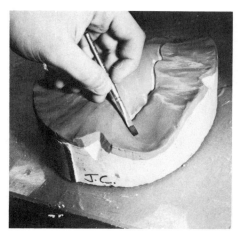

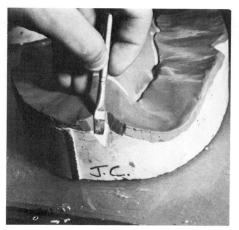

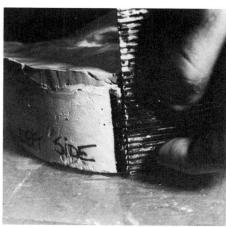

15. Now the modeled piece must be cast. First apply a thin layer of sealer or cap material all over the clay model and overflow. This should be done very carefully so that you don't ruin the textures. (If you are worried about the textures, this step isn't essential, but the sealer does keep the clay from sticking to the negative. You can always add more texture after you have applied the sealer.)

16. You can apply the same material sparingly over the keys. Or use petroleum jelly in the keys.

17. Place one end of a strip of rubber matting next to the mark of the original rubber strip on the side of the mold.

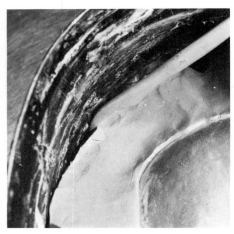

18. Wrap it around and secure it with masking tape.

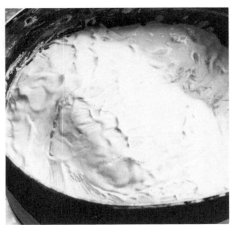

19. If you executed steps 12 and 13 correctly, the clay should touch the rubber wall all the way around.

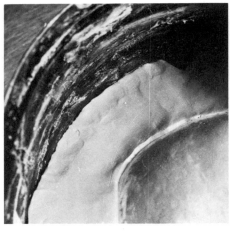

20. If it doesn't, either press the clay with your fingers to make it touch the wall, or roll a bit of clay, place it between the clay surface and the rubber wall, and fill the gap.

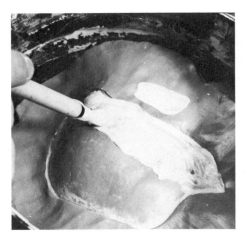

21. Mix a small amount of plaster (Ultracal 30 or B-11). Make sure it contains no air bubbles and that it is very smooth and creamy. It is *essential* to use a brush to apply the first couple of layers. Make sure the first layer has set before you apply the second, and rinse the brush between applications.

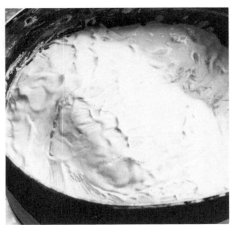

22. Gently cover the entire surface of the mold with plaster.

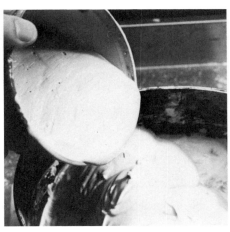

23. While these two layers are setting, mix a larger batch of plaster and remove the air bubbles by hitting the bowl on the table. Gently pour the plaster into the mold from one side and let it spread by itself, so that no air bubbles can get trapped underneath. If you are using wire reinforcement in the mold, insert it now (see Chapter Two).

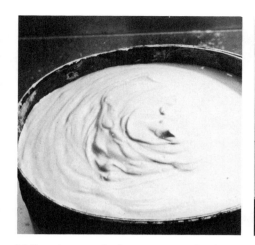

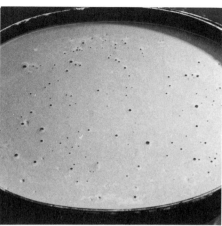

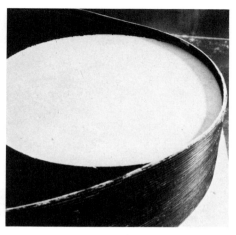

24. Pour in enough plaster to cover the tip of the wire reinforcement by about ½ inch (13 mm). If you are not using the reinforcement, mark the inside of the rubber wall 1 inch (25 mm) or so above the highest point of the mold or the modeling, whichever is higher, and pour in the plaster to there.

25. If the mold is on a board, hold the board and gently rock it back and forth. If the mold is not on a board, gently move the mold itself back and forth. This smooths the plaster on top and raises trapped air bubbles to the surface.

26. Wait for the plaster to go through its chemical changes, first hot, then cold. When it is totally dry, remove the rubber wall. (If you open the mold while the plaster is still hot, you will find soft clay inside.)

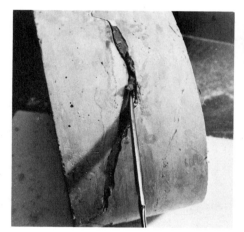

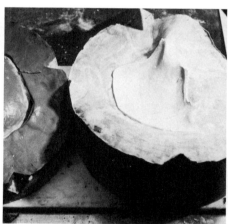

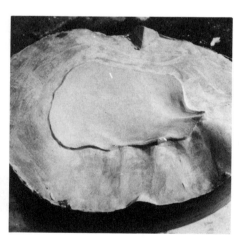

27. To open the mold, place it on its side, and with the aid of a tool gently separate the two halves.

28. The clay has not stuck to the negative because sealer or cap material was used. If you don't use it, because you are afraid of ruining the texture, and the clay sticks to the negative, you can clean it with alcohol and cotton, and possibly a stiff brush, depending on the mold and its texture.

29. This is the negative of the modeled piece. Before removing the clay from the positive, clean off the sealer or cap material with cotton and acetone; then remove the clay and clean the mold with cotton and alcohol.

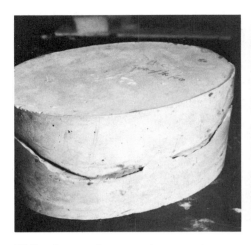

30. Put the two pieces together, negative at the bottom and positive on the top. The space between the molds, where the clay was, is now empty, ready for the foam.

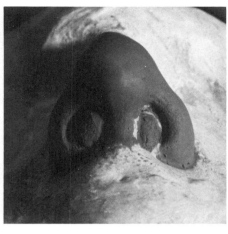

1. After the crude modeling of the nose is placed over the positive, finish the modeling and fill the nostrils if they are deep-set.

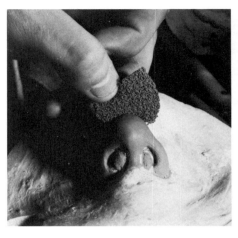

2. Texture the nose with red rubber sponge or orange peel, whichever is appropriate for the character.

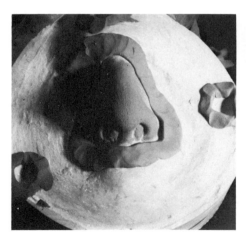

3. Create a cutting edge around the nose and the keys.

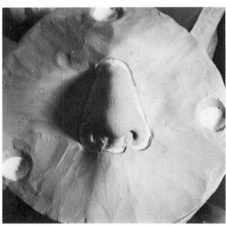

4. Add clay to create the overflow.

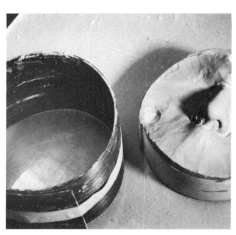

5. To cast the nose, place a rubber-matting wall around the model and secure it with masking tape. Then remove the wall and put it aside.

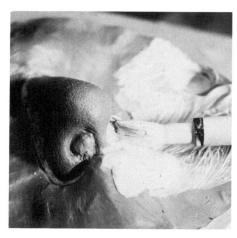

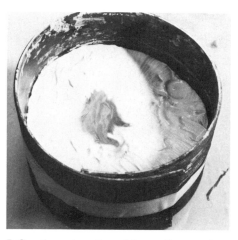

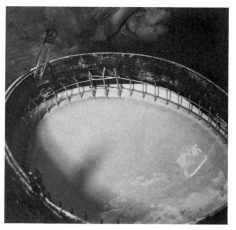

6. Mix a very small amount of plaster, and make sure it has no air bubbles in it. Brush on the first couple of layers while the mold is *outside* the rubber wall (it is easier to get to the nostrils that way).

7. Gently replace the rubber wall around the mold.

8. If you are using wire reinforcement, add it now. Don't push the wire down to penetrate the clay under it. Gently let it sit over the first couple of layers of plaster.

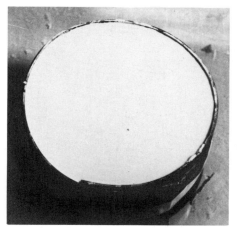

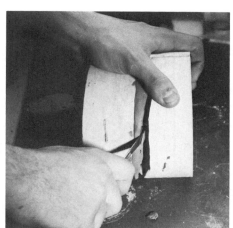

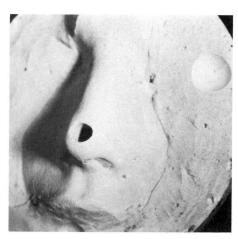

9. While the first two layers of plaster are setting, mix a larger batch. Gently pour it inside the mold from one side and let it spread to fill the mold to about 1 inch (25 mm) above the tip of the nose. Rock the board under the mold to smooth out the plaster and remove trapped air bubbles.

10. When the plaster is totally dry, remove the rubber wall. Place the mold on its side and separate the two sections.

11. Clean both sides, and then drill a ¼-inch (6-mm) escape hole in the positive, where the thickest part of the foam will be. You can determine that by remembering the modeling. In this case the very tip of the nose is the thickest. You can drill more than one hole in a given mold, provided you know where the thickest parts are. (The escape holes allow excess foam latex to flow out.)

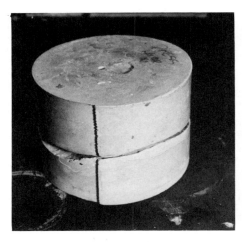

12. Place the positive and the negative together, and the mold is ready for the foam latex.

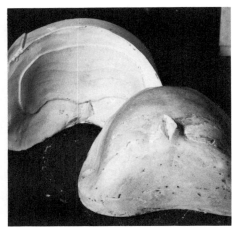

13. When the forehead and chin have been made, all the small pieces are ready.

MODELING AND CASTING HANDS

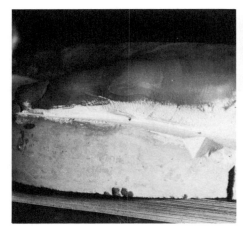

1. In the modeling of hands you will run up against more undercuts than you can imagine. Each finger has an undercut all around it, where the sides of the fingers begin to curve under. Mark these areas with pencil before you begin your modeling, and make sure you don't go below that line. In fact, stay slightly above it.

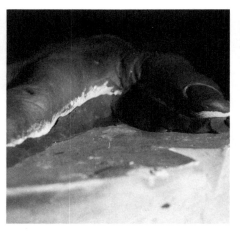

2. After the modeling is done and the thin edges are modeled, add the clay for the cutting edge. Keep it as close to the edge of the modeling as you can. The cutting edge should end where the fingers begin to curve under.

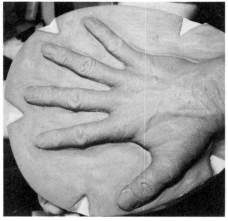

3. Spread the clay to the edge of the mold to build the overflow. At this time, as for other modeled pieces, cover the hand, including the keys, with a thin coat of sealer or cap material, or coat the keys with petroleum jelly.

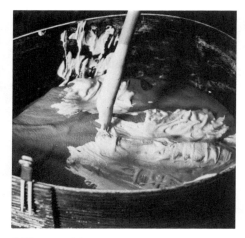

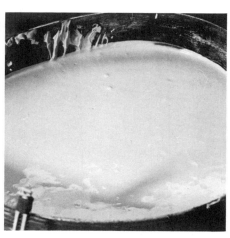

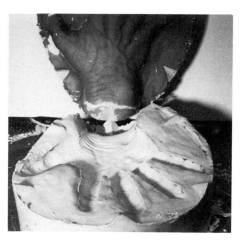

4. Place a rubber wall around the mold and mix a smooth, creamy batch of plaster. Get rid of the air bubbles and brush on the first couple of layers.

5. While the first layers are setting, mix a larger batch of plaster. Pour it inside the mold from the wrist or the palm of the hand and let it spread by itself to fill the fingers and the mold. Allow the plaster to dry totally.

6. Remove the rubber wall and separate the parts of the mold. If there are no undercuts, the mold will open easily; otherwise, forget it—you will have to start over.

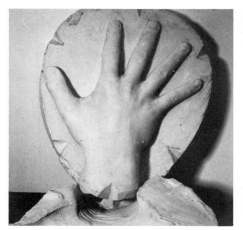

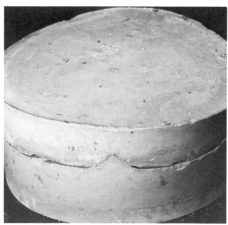

7. Clean the clay with acetone to take off the sealer. Then remove the clay and clean the mold and all its crevices with a brush and alcohol, if necessary.

8. Put the two pieces together. The mold is now ready for the foam. (We have cast only one of the subject's hands; make sure you cast both.)

CHAPTER EIGHT

MODELING AND CASTING LARGE PIECES

In the preceding chapter we explained the technique of preparing small pieces. Some of them were designed for the subject at age forty; others will be used for the next age, fifty-five. Here we are going to finish the modeling and casting for three-quarters of the face and the full face.

■ MATERIALS AND EQUIPMENT ■

Clay

Modeling tools

Three ¾-inch (19-mm) brushes

Sealer or cap material

Petroleum jelly

Plaster (Ultracal 30 or B-11)

Japanese brush

Spatula

Burlap

Scissors

Surgical knife

Electric or hand drill and ¾-inch (19-mm) bit 6 inches (15 cm) long

Acetone

Alcohol

Cotton

Acrylic or wooden board

Surform tool

Latex stamps

MODELING THREE-QUARTERS OF THE FACE

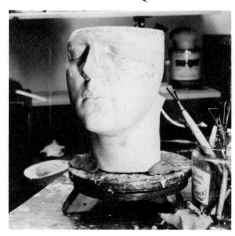

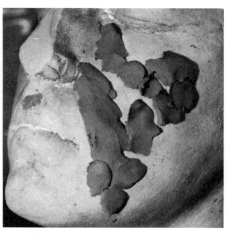

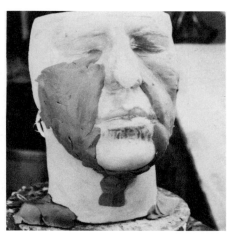

1. Place the positive of the subject's life mask either on a modeling stand that has a turntable, or if you prefer, prop it upright on your worktable. You must be able to move the positive around to different lighting sources to examine the shape and smoothness of the modeling. (An overhead and a side light together or individually will help you.)

2. Begin by applying small pieces of clean clay over the area to be modeled. In this case it is the sides of the face and under the chin and neck combined.

3. Use your fingers to spread the clay, creating thickness where you need it and thin areas where they will give the piece the proper muscle structure for the character and his age. As you model, remember the undercuts, the relationship between the modeled sections and the rest of the face, and, of course, the subject's own muscle structure.

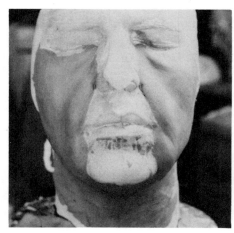

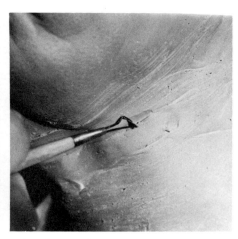

4. Select modeling tools to remove extra clay, to smooth the surface of the modeling, and to get into corners where your fingers cannot reach.

5. Continue until you have finished the face. You must be extremely careful with the outside edges of the piece. No matter how thick the piece is, no matter how small or large it is, you must taper it to the edges until it is very thin. The thinner the better; otherwise you will wind up with a foam-latex piece with thick edges, which will make it obvious to the naked eye as well as the camera that it is not the subject's own skin.

Depending on how good you are, how fast you work, and how much of a perfectionist you are, it might take anywhere from a few hours to a few days to finish a piece. It is very difficult for an artist to let go of his work, but at some point you must put down your tools and say, "This is it." Otherwise, you can keep going forever trying to improve your work.

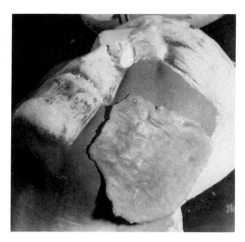 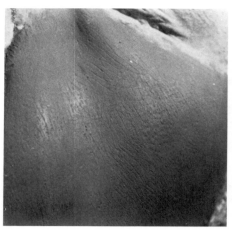 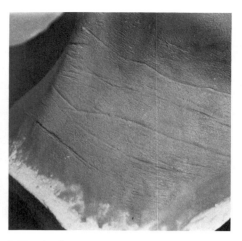

6. Select a latex stamp appropriate for the piece you have just finished. Place it over the clay model and press it down.

7. You can create most natural-looking skin textures.

8. For the lines of the neck, select the stamp that can best create what you need. Because of the size of the latex stamps, you must go over the clay model section by section. Make sure the lines, both large and small, fall in the proper place and maintain continuity.

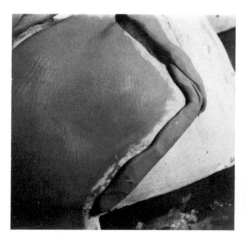 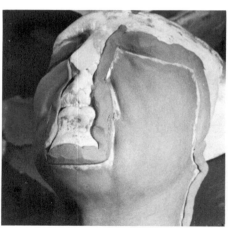 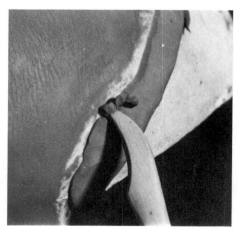

9. As was explained for small pieces in Chapter Seven, very carefully roll a small piece of clay to create the cutting edge all around the piece, about ¼ inch (6 mm) from the edge of the modeling.

10. Gently press the clay down to adhere it to the life mask. At the same time move it closer to the edges by about ⅛ inch (3 mm).

11. With a wooden tool cut the edge of the clay nearest the modeling. Make the edge as shallow as you can.

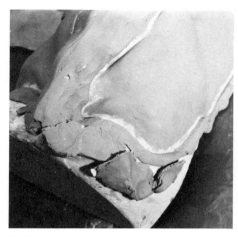

12. Cover the rest of the exposed plaster with clay, and extend the cutting edge to the edge of the mold for the overflow.

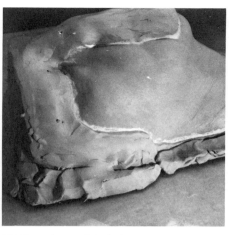

13. Place the modeled piece on a board and secure it with used clay as shown.

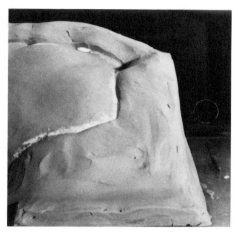

14. Make the bottom of the mold wider than the top. This will facilitate opening it later on.

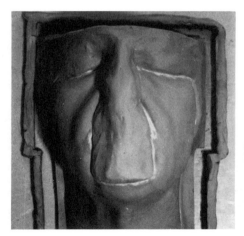

15. Build a low clay wall about 1 inch (25 mm) high all around the mold and about 1½ inches (4 cm) away from it.

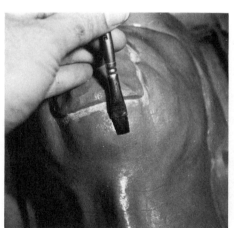

16. To make sure that the clay model will not stick to the negative, cover the entire model with a thin coat of liquid plastic sealer or cap material. Apply it very carefully and in a thin coat or it will fill all your texturing lines.

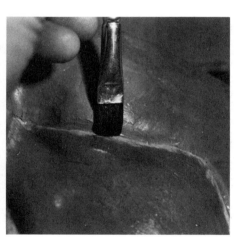

17. Since this material will act as a separating agent, you can use it over the keys if there are any.

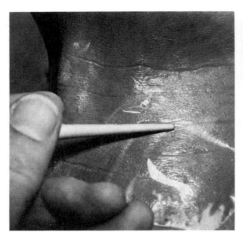 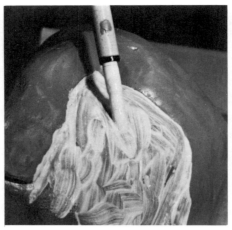 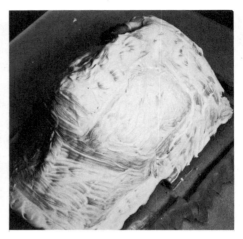

18. This is your last chance to make changes in or additions to your work. If you want to add extra lines or wrinkles, place cellophane paper over the clay (if you have not applied sealer) and add them with modeling tools. Sealer functions like cellophane paper, so if you have used it you can add lines directly.

19. Mix a small amount of plaster (Ultracal 30 or B-11). Make sure there are no air bubbles trapped under the surface by gently hitting the bowl on the table. With a Japanese brush apply a thin coat all over the piece. Concentrate on the modeled areas and the cutting edges only. To make sure there are no air bubbles trapped anywhere, bend over the mold and blow over the wet plaster to move it around (see step 5, page 21).

20. Allow the first layer to set partially, when it does not look wet and shiny anymore.

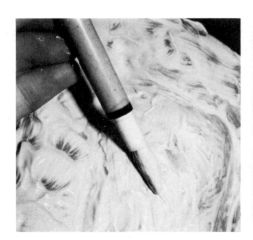 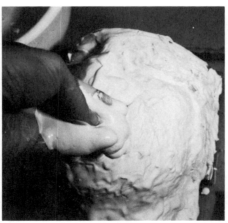 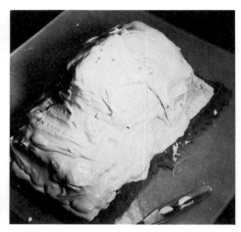

21. Add the second layer of plaster in the same way, without disturbing the first layer. (Rinse the brush in clean water after each use.)

22. While the second layer is setting, mix a larger batch of plaster and eliminate the air bubbles. Gently apply the plaster over the first two layers with your hand. Make sure you do not accidentally touch the surface of the mold. Just pour the plaster on the very top and let it slide down the sides. This decreases the chances that air bubbles will get trapped.

23. Continue adding plaster until it is at least ½ inch (13 mm) thick all over. Make sure that the plaster stays inside the clay wall around the mold.

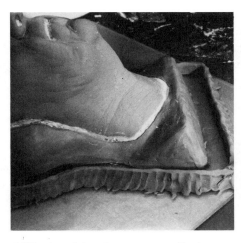

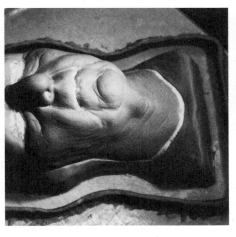

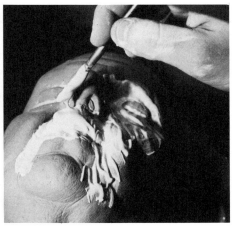

6. We placed the piece on an acrylic sheet and built a short wall around it.

7. Molds of this shape do not need keys. First of all, there is no room for them. Second, the two pieces fit together as if there were invisible keys here and there. You may add them if you think it's necessary, however.

8. We mixed a batch of plaster and applied the first couple of layers with a brush.

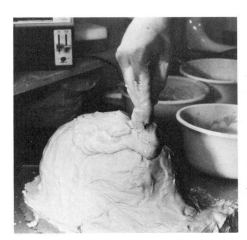

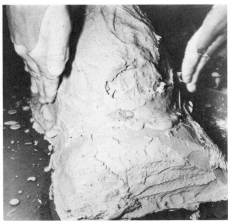

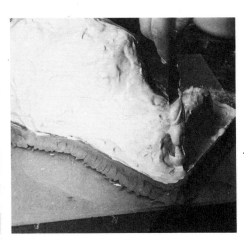

9. Then we added enough plaster to build the thickness to about ¼ inch (6 mm).

10. We reinforced the mold with burlap and smoothed it out with a spatula.

11. Then we covered the reinforcement with additional plaster.

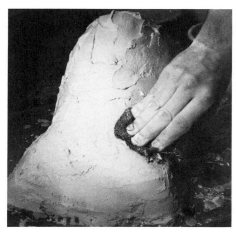

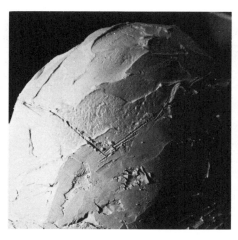

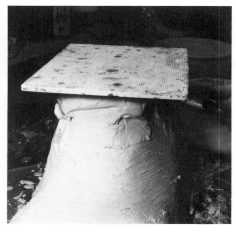

12. While the plaster was setting, we smoothed the surface with a wet piece of burlap.

13. To create a base for the mold, we marked the top.

14. Then we spread a batch of plaster heavily on the very top and pressed a sheet of milk glass onto it. (A sheet of plastic could also be used.) We filled and smoothed under it, then left it alone to dry.

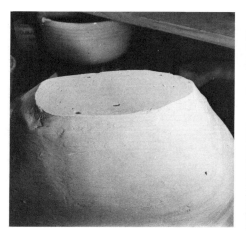

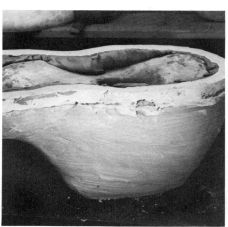

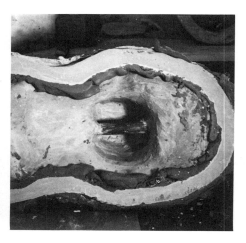

15. After removing the milk glass, we did a little doctoring to get the base clean and smooth.

16. We turned the mold upside down and placed it on its base.

17. At this stage the mold consisted of an outer shell and a narrow clay section separating the outer shell from the positive in the center.

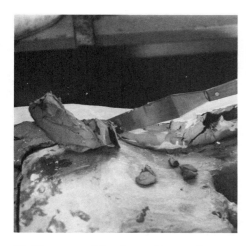

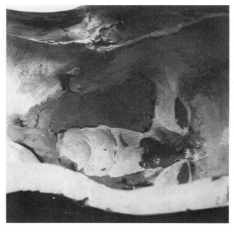

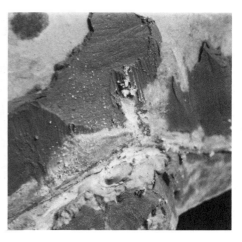

18. We removed the clay and began the separation process with anticipation and apprehension. We pulled the mold, sat on it, used a hammer and chisel—and it did not open. Though we thought we had taken care to avoid undercuts, one or two were nevertheless preventing the molds from separating. When we finally pried them apart, they were damaged.

19. Because we had not used sealer on the clay model, most of the clay stuck to the negative mold.

20. We discovered undercuts near the ear on either side of the mold. Pulling scraped the negative and the positive here, . . .

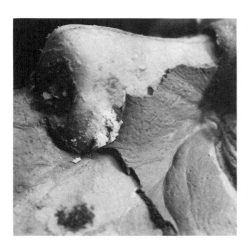

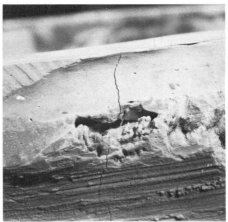

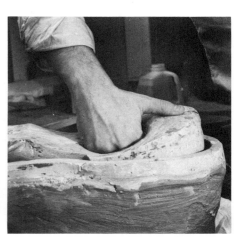

21. . . . and on the outside of the nostrils.

22. The result was a big crack on the negative mold all the way along the side of the face and neck. The cracked mold was held together only by the burlap reinforcement. We should have thrown out this negative and started over. But we decided to see what would happen if we mended the mold and ran through a batch of foam. (This might happen if you're running short of time.)

23. We cleaned both molds, then put them together to see how much pressure was needed to lock the molds without further damage.

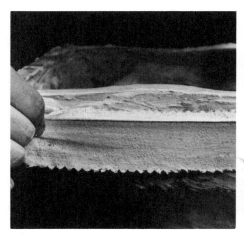

24. To make sure that the crack would not open wider in the heat of the oven, we wrapped a few layers of plaster bandage and Celastic around it.

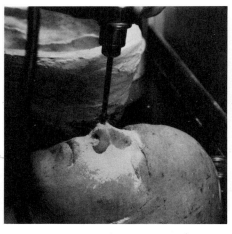

25. Because of the size of the mold, we drilled two escape holes in the positive where the foam was thickest, one over the nose.

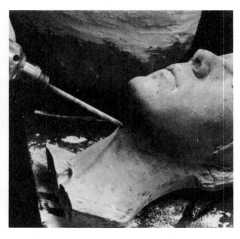

26. We made another at the neck.

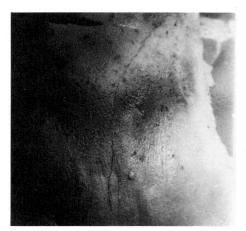

27. We mixed a batch of foam latex for a test. (The complete process for using foam latex is explained in Chapter Nine.) The result was a piece of foam latex that reproduced the crack on the mold. Our mistake is proof of the difficulty undercuts can cause, and it demonstrates why you must be careful to avoid them. We threw out the damaged mold.

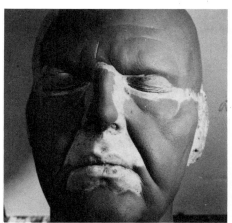

28. We began the modeling again, this time remembering the undercuts as well as the relationship of this age to the others.

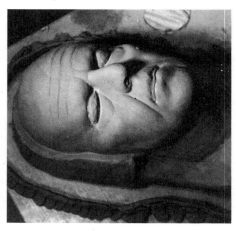

29. As before, we placed the modeled piece on an acrylic sheet and built a short clay wall around it.

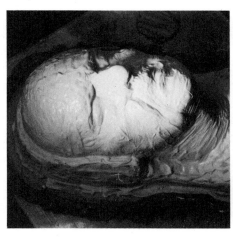

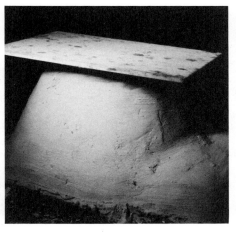

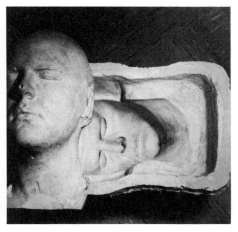

30. We mixed a batch of plaster and applied the first couple of layers with a brush.

31. We added reinforcement and placed milk glass on top of the mold, then added plaster to create a flat base.

32. This time the mold separated without any trouble.

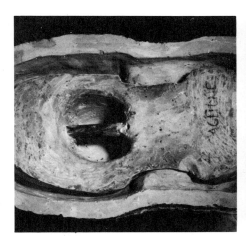

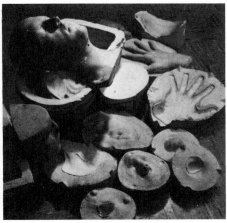

33. We cleaned the negative and positive to get them ready for the foam latex.

34. Here are the numerous molds made for the gradual aging of our subject.

The next step is making the foam latex. In the case of gradual aging it is absolutely necessary that one person do all the modeling. If more people are involved, extreme cooperation and exact understanding of the relationship between the pieces is vital. As we have said before, it is better to finish all the pieces before casting any.

REINFORCING A FOAM-RUBBER MASK

If you have to make a foam-rubber mask for a show where it will be used night after night and will not be glued to the actor's face, you can make the entire mask by brushing eight to ten layers of latex inside the negative and reinforcing it with cheese-cloth or muslin towels. Or you can make the mask from foam rubber to fit the actor's face and reinforce it with a pair of ladies' panty hose:

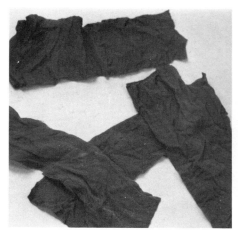

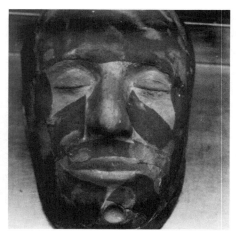

1. Cut off the legs of the panty hose and divide the upper part into small sections.

2. Glue these sections with liquid latex, as adhesive, over the thick parts of the positive mold. (Do not use any other adhesive; it will not work.) You should know where the thick parts of the molded piece are. Then follow the process of making foam (explained in Chapter Nine).

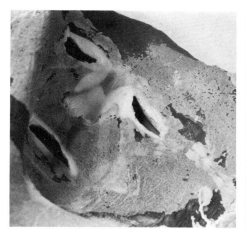

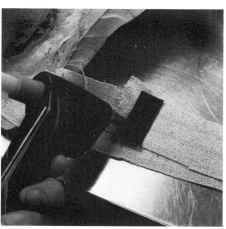

3. When the foam is ready and the molds are separated, the material shows through the back of the piece.

4. If you have to attach straps to the mask to be fastened over the head, use hot glue and Velcro for easy adjustment.

PART THREE:

MAKING AND APPLYING FOAM LATEX

CHAPTER NINE
FOAM LATEX

Foam latex, the material used to make the final prosthetic pieces, comes in liquid form. Each manufacturer has its own formula:

George Bau's has four ingredients: latex, curing agent, foaming agent, and jelling agent.

Uniroyal Chemical recommends a four-part formula: latex, sulfur dispersion, zinc-oxide dispersion, and jelling agent.

Kryolan has a three-part formula known as Foam System "Compound Hagen." This is a cold procedure technique; that is, it does not require baking.

Paramount offers a three-part formula.

Of these, G. Bau's formula makes the softest foam, and most makeup artists use it for the face where a thick and flexible structure is required.

The simplest formula that produces a good-quality foam is R and D foam latex. It has only three ingredients: latex (Part A), curing paste (Part B), and jelling agent (Part C). R and D is what we have used to create the makeup in this book, and that is the kind we are going to explain how to use. This procedure does not work for other kinds of foam. All of them have special instructions on each bottle or jar which must be followed exactly for best results. (My experience tells me, however, that at times you must forget the manufacturer's instructions and change the formula to suit your immediate need, such as when you want the foam to jell slower or faster, or when you want it to be softer or harder.)

MATERIALS AND EQUIPMENT

R and D foam latex

Electric mixer

Spiral stirrer

Balance scale or equivalent

Stainless-steel measuring beaker

Oven

Pocket stopwatch and/or clock

Wooden stick, chopstick, or plastic swizzle stick marked with gradations up to 5 or 6 inches (12 to 15 cm)

Thermometer (room temperature will affect the quality of the foam)

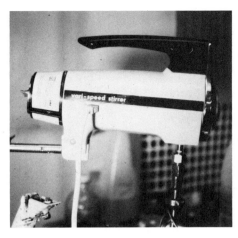

This electric mixer is called a "Vari Speed Stirrer," designed to be mounted for easy adjustment of height. It has speeds of 1 to 12 and a single stirrer. You could also use a Sunbeam electric mixer with two beaters. (Take one of them out, or replace them with something more suitable, as we have.)

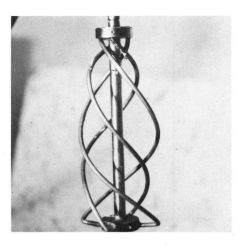

This spiral stirrer has been specially designed for easy access to the corners of the vessel to mix all the ingredients evenly. You cannot buy it anywhere; it must be custom-made.

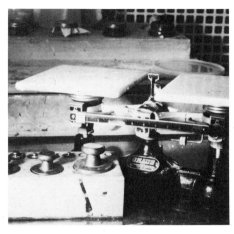

For accurate measurement of all the compounds you need a scale to weigh from 1 gram to at least 1,600 grams. Use the kind that you balance with weights on two plates, or with counterweights on a bar. (Instead you can use measuring cups and spoons.)

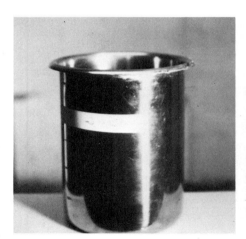

A stainless-steel vessel about 6 inches (15 cm) in diameter by 8 inches (20½ cm) high is good for the normal-size batch of foam. A mixing bowl or plastic container the same size can also serve the purpose.

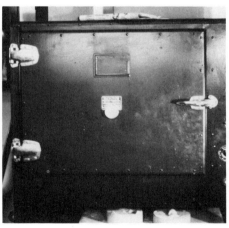

To be able to bake and cure the foam, you must have an oven large enough to hold at least eight to ten small molds or fewer large ones. You must be able to control the temperature of the oven. If you use a kitchen oven, get a dial-type oven thermometer and leave it next to the molds. Check it often to make sure the temperature is right.

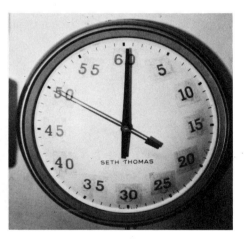

Instead of a pocket stopwatch, you can convert a regular clock for easy reading. Change the hours to minutes by covering the numbers on the clock face with numbers cut out from a wall calendar. Paint the hour hand to camouflage it. A switch somewhere on the cord will help you turn the clock off and on as you need. It is a good idea to have both a clock and a stopwatch.

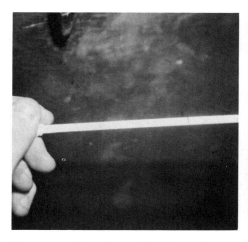

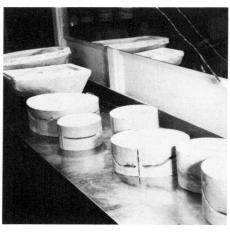

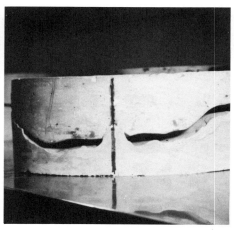

To measure the volume of the foam after beating it, you can use a piece of clean, smooth wood, a chopstick, or a plastic swizzle stick marked like a ruler up to 5 or 6 inches (12 to 15 cm). You insert this into the foam to see how high it has risen. (The higher the foam, the softer and more flexible the prosthetic pieces will be.)

1. On a table near where you will mix the latex, line up the molds with all the negatives on the bottom and all the positives on top.

2. With a marking pen draw one or two vertical lines from the top mold (the positive) to the lower mold (the negative).

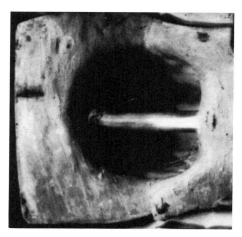

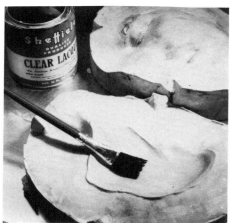

"R and D foam is not like some others for which castor oil or silicone is the usual separator," reports makeup artist Dick Smith. "The calcium in the gypsum affects the R and D foam, causing it to collapse into larger bubbles. It requires a separator that seals the surface. One coat of clear lacquer or two coats of diluted lacquer work very well and will last for many bakings. Be sure first to clean the molds thoroughly with acetone to get rid of all the grease. Instead of lacquer, a stearic acid separator may be used. A separator called Seporal may be used even over the lacquer separator to make the removal of the appliances even easier."

3. In larger molds in which the positive falls in place easily, it is still wise to mark the top of both molds for easy and precise placement of the positive.

4. To separate the molds without difficulty and without damaging the foam after they are out of the oven, each manufacturer suggests a separating agent.

MEASURING AND MIXING THE FOAM LATEX

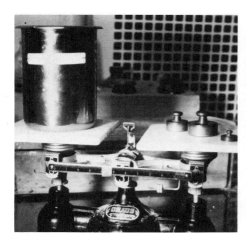

5. Place all the positives behind their corresponding negatives, preferably on their sides.

There are two things you must do before anything else:

First, turn the oven on. It will be at the proper temperature by the time the molds are ready. Because the oven is empty at first, it will get warm fast and the temperature will rise above what you need. The best temperature is 210° F. (99° C.). When you put the molds in the oven, you will lose some heat, and it will take longer for the temperature to rise again because the molds are cold and absorb some of the heat. The smaller and fewer the molds, the faster the oven heats up. After half an hour or so, however, the heat in the oven should be steady.

The second item to remember and check is the temperature of the room, which affects the jelling of the foam. At a temperature below 70° F. (21° C.) it might not jell at all; if you change the formula and add more jelling agent, it might jell too fast.

When the temperature is above 80° F. (27° C.), the foam will be very lumpy. If you beat the foam more than is necessary in order to get greater volume, it will jell faster. The best jelling time is between 8 and 10 minutes. (You can delay the jelling time to more than 10 minutes if you have to by decreasing the amount of jelling agent or adding a few drops of ammonia.) The best temperature is between 68° and 72° F. (20° to 22° C.).

It is a good idea to keep a log. Write down everything you do and every step you take, and describe any variations you use. Include these data: date, room temperature, grams used of Part A and Part B, beating time, volume, refining time, grams used of jelling agent (Part C), mixing time, jelling time, baking time, and the result. This information will help you to understand the nature of your work and how to solve problems when they arise.

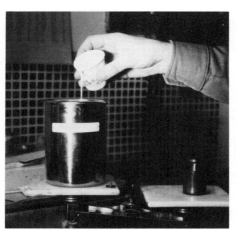

1. Shake all the ingredients well. Place the empty mixing vessel on the scale and put enough weight on the opposite side to balance it. Add another 170 grams. This is the amount of latex recommended by the R and D Latex Corporation for one batch.

2. Gently pour 170 grams of Part A (latex) into the empty vessel until the two sides of the scale balance. This will be easier if you first pour the latex from the gallon-size container into a small paper cup.

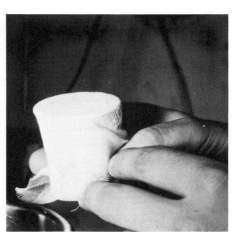

3. If the latex is not smooth, stretch a piece of cheesecloth over the paper cup and squeeze the cup over the vessel.

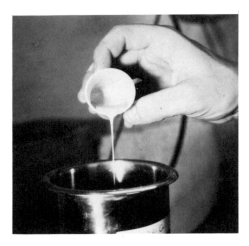

4. Add 22 grams of weight to the scale, bringing the total to 192 grams. Then pour 22 grams of Part B (curing paste) into a small plastic or waxed-paper cup and very gently add that to the mixing vessel. You cannot remove any excess, so you must be extremely careful to add no more than 22 grams.

If you don't have a scale, measure 7 fluid ounces of Part A, 1 level tablespoon of Part B, and 1 level teaspoon of Part C, filled till it overflows. A level teaspoon is about 8 grams. If the first batch is not jelled in 15 minutes, use 1½ teaspoons (12 grams) in the next batch.

To prevent sticking, clean the rims of all the jars, place a piece of plastic wrap on top, and then screw on the caps.

You can add color to the latex now, before beating it, or add it later, mixed with the jelling agent (Part C). It is not at all necessary to color foam latex, because it will be colored after application; but it is easier to work with colored appliances. If you add color to the jelling agent and mix it in the vessel, you will be able to tell whether

the jelling agent is mixed uniformly.

For a light flesh tone, mix ½ teaspoon of burnt sienna casein and ¼ teaspoon of water. For dark flesh tones use 1 teaspoon of color to ½ teaspoon of water. There are other colors, such as Universal Colorint and Tints-All (see list of supplies). There is no set formula for it; each makeup artist prefers certain shades. You must mix these colors, do some testing, and find out your own formula for the right face. Keep records of all the mixtures and the results. They will help you choose the right one for the right skin tone.

If you want to add the color without the jelling agent, simply pour the mixture or drops into the vessel now, before beating.

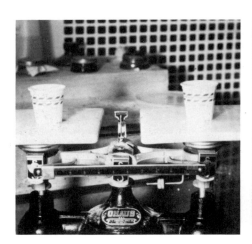

5. If you are going to mix the color with the jelling agent, take everything off the scale and place a small waxed or plastic cup on each side. Or put a cup on one side and balance it with an equal amount of weight on the other side.

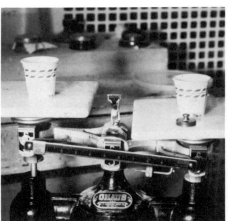

6. Add 9 grams of weight to one side of the scale.

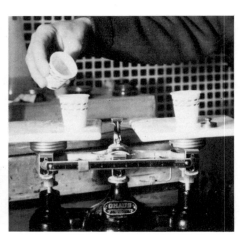

7. Gently pour 9 grams of jelling agent (Part C) into the other cup to balance the scale. (Pour some out of the original jar into a cup and from there into the cup on the scale.)

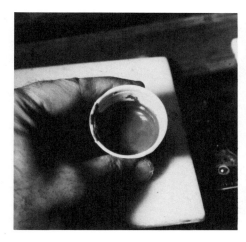

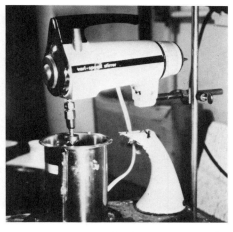

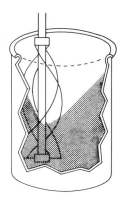

8. Add the coloring mixture to the jelling agent and mix them well. Set the mixture aside until you are ready for it. I prefer to prepare Part C and the color later, while the foam is being refined. The first few times, however, you might get rushed and panicky, so it is better to prepare the mixture ahead of time.

9. Place the vessel under the mixer. If at all possible, adjust the stirrer so that it is at one side of the vessel instead of in the center.

10. Before we continue, let us examine a cross section of the vessel to see what happens when the latex is beaten. At the highest speed of the mixer, the latex creeps up the sides of the vessel before it reaches the proper volume, or height. If you are not careful, it will fly out of the container and splatter the work area and you as well.

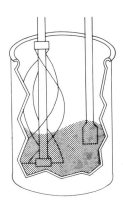

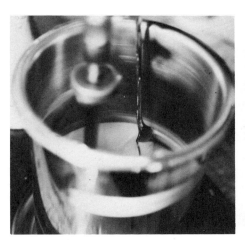

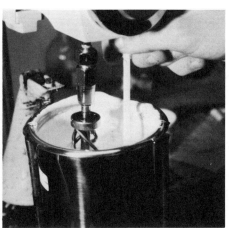

11. At the same high speed, however, a long spoon or narrow rubber spatula inside the vessel, just touching the walls, will do two things: (a) prevent the latex from rising to the top before it is foamed, and (b) direct the liquid toward the center of the stirrer and make it foam faster. You must hold the spoon or spatula at all times and move it upward as the foam rises, keeping the head of the spatula or the bowl of the spoon at the top of the liquid.

12. Start the stopwatch, set the mixer at its highest speed, and turn it on. Make sure the mixing vessel or bowl spins slowly under the fast-rotating stirrer. Depending on your mixer, its speed, your experience, and other conditions, the 1 inch (25 mm) of liquid in the vessel will foam up in 2 to 6 minutes.

13. To measure the volume, turn off the mixer, stop the stopwatch, and insert the measuring stick in the vessel.

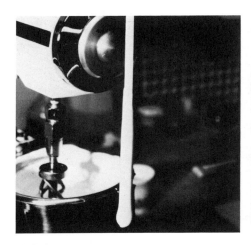

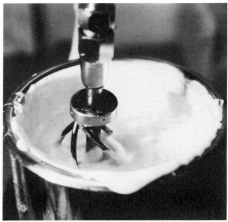

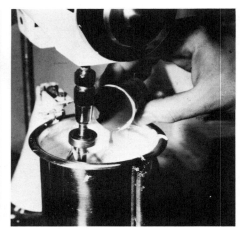

14. Take out the stick to see how far the latex has foamed up. If it is not high enough, start the clock and the mixer and beat the latex a few minutes longer until it reaches the desired height. For a while you will have to stop and go until you get used to the work. The best volume for soft R and D foam is about 4 to 4½ inches (10 to 12 cm).

15. When the right volume is reached, lower the mixer speed to 3, check the clock, and let the mixer run slowly for 3 to 4 minutes. This process is called "refining"; it breaks all the large air bubbles in the foam.

16. Then, while the mixer is still spinning at low speed, pour the jelling agent (Part C) and color directly into the center of the foam. (If you have already added the color, just add the jelling agent.) Use a spoon to get every drop out of the cup and into the mixing vessel.

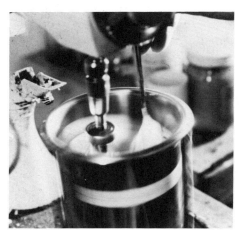

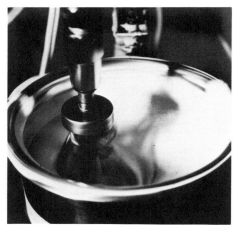

17. Insert a narrow spatula or spoon in the vessel, as before, and while the mixer and the vessel spin, help mix the jelling agent and color with the foam. Do not do this too vigorously or you will add too much air to the foam. After 1 minute the contents of the vessel should be evenly colored, which means the jelling agent has been mixed uniformly. Be sure to get the spatula or spoon to the very bottom of the vessel and into the corners to mix the color thoroughly.

18. Take out the spoon or spatula and run the mixer for no longer than another minute. At the end of this time the foam is ready to be poured into the molds. It is a good idea to put the second stopwatch on as soon as you begin to pour the jelling agent into the vessel and stop it when the foam is jelled. Write the jelling time in your log. After a few times you will be able to decide how you can speed up or slow down the jelling time according to your needs.

FILLING AND CURING THE MOLDS

If you need to fill more than four or five small molds, have someone help you, at least at first; one person fills them and the other closes them. When you have more experience, you will develop your own system and be able to handle the job by yourself. Beginners tend to rush through this step because they are not sure how soon the foam will jell. Sometimes it jells after the first mold is filled; sometimes it takes more than 15 or 20 minutes. Sometimes the foam jells in the vessel; sometimes it does not jell at all. Take your time; it is better to fill a few molds successfully than all the molds badly.

Another problem is how much foam is necessary for each mold. The tendency is to pour in a lot, but this runs off and fills all the keys, resulting in thick edges on the appliances which usually make them unusable. Again, it takes experience to know how much foam to use. The rule to follow is really very simple. Just remember how much clay you used to model the piece and how thick it was—that is how much foam you need.

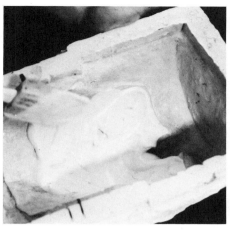

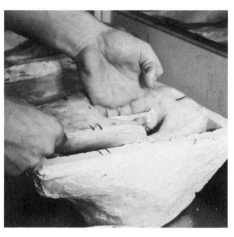

1. Use a large rubber spatula for large molds and a small one for small molds. For large molds, slide the foam out of the vessel into the negative mold, preferably at the side, and spread it all over the modeled area, making sure that in your haste you do not trap any air bubbles under the foam in the folds and crevices. If a nose is included in the large mold, use a small amount of foam and work it from the bridge to the tip.

2. When the large mold is filled, place the positive mold on top and align the pen marks.

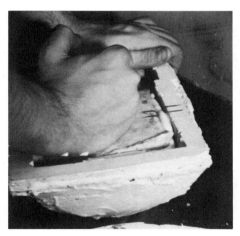

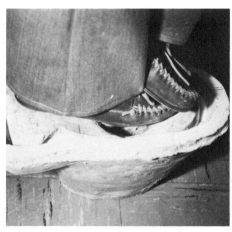

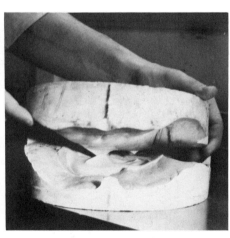

3. Let the positive slide gently inside the negative. Help it by pressing.

4. When the positive is in place, put the mold on the floor and stand on it. Don't be afraid to put all your weight on it.

5. The procedure is the same for small molds; use a small spatula. Pour a small amount of foam inside the negative and make sure all the deeply textured areas and deep crevices are filled. Place the positive on top with the pen marks aligned on the side of the molds and gently close them.

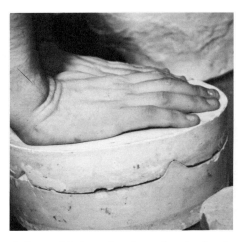

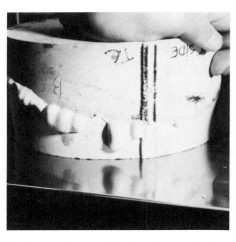

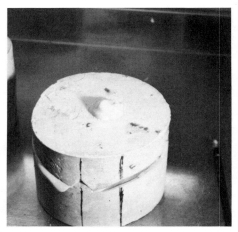

6. Press with the palm of your hand as hard as you can. *Do not* clamp the molds and *do not* reopen them after they are closed.

7. Now you must wait. If you have mixed the foam with care and followed the procedure correctly, the foam latex will jell. How do you know when it has? With your fingertip press the foam at the sides of the molds.

8. Or press the foam that has escaped from the escape holes on the top.

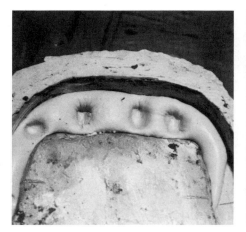

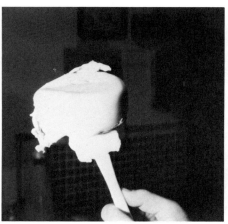

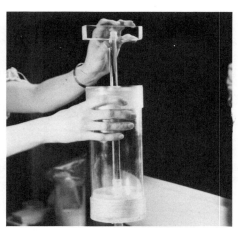

9. Or check the overflow foam around the large mold. If no liquid comes out, and your finger leaves a deep impression in the foam, it has jelled.

10. If some foam is left in the mixing vessel, pull out the spatula; if the foam has jelled, it will be attached to the spatula. Check the stopwatch and mark the time in your log. If the foam does not jell in 15 minutes, it will start to break down and may collapse altogether. (See steps 27–29, pages 109–110, for what to do in such a case.)

11. Another way of filling a mold is by injecting the foam into the mold through an escape hole with an injection gun. I don't think this technique is necessary for small molds. You can use it if you want to. It certainly has its advantages in large molds.

To begin with, for a large mold you must make a couple of tests to find out how much foam you actually need; you may need a larger vessel. When the foam is ready, pour it inside the gun and squeeze it through. How can you tell when the mold is filled? Wherever possible, without damaging the foam piece, drill escape holes, which allow the air to escape as the foam fills the mold. When foam comes out of each hole, you can tell how far you have to go. Of course, as you pass each hole you must plug it; otherwise the foam will keep pouring out instead of filling the mold. You must squeeze slowly, and you must calculate the time so that the foam does not jell when you are only halfway through. You might need someone to help you by handing you another injector with more foam if necessary.

As for the injection gun itself, you cannot buy it anywhere. You must get all the pieces and make one, or have it made for you.

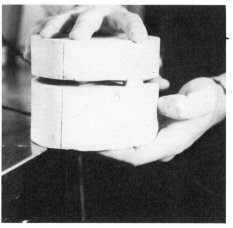

12. By this time the oven should be heated. During the process of putting the molds in the oven, do not leave the oven door open; close it after you have put each mold in. Handle the molds one at a time and with extreme care. It is better to slide each mold from the table to your hand instead of lifting it. If the distance between the oven and where the molds are is more than 10 or 12 feet (3 to 4 m), first move all the molds as close to the oven as you can.

How long should the molds be in the oven? The usual time for a two-piece mold about 4 inches (10 cm) high, 2 inches (5 cm) for each side, is 2 to 2½ hours at 210° F. (99° C.). Larger pieces require more time, depending on their size and how fresh they are. You must watch the oven temperature and regulate it until it settles down to the proper setting. Then leave it alone. A good way to keep track of the time is to attach a piece of paper to the oven and write on it the time you put the molds in and the time they should come out.

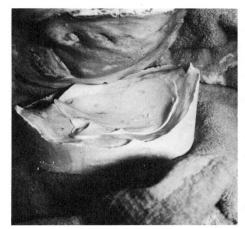

13. When it is time to take the molds out, you must make sure the foam is cured. Take one mold out with a hand towel.

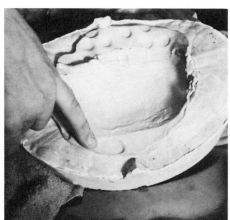

14. If there is a piece of foam on the side or on the top of the mold, press it with your finger. If the foam snaps back like a piece of rubber, it is cured. It is even better to open the mold gently and perform the same test on the piece inside, but *not* on the usable sections; touch only the overflow areas. If the foam shows your finger mark, it is not yet cured. In that case *do not* close the mold; return the side with the foam attached to it to the oven for another half hour.

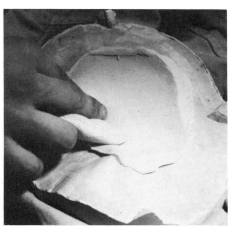

15. If your test shows that the foam is cured, powder the foam piece.

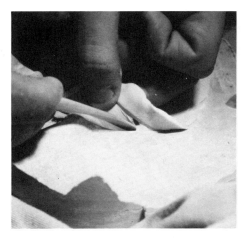

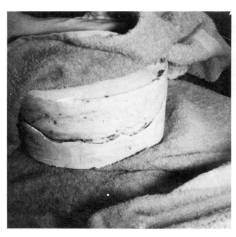

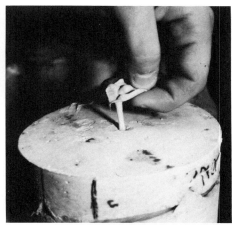

16. Now very gently remove the foam. Be extremely careful not to tear or damage the thin edges. You can use small wooden tools or a small brush dipped in powder to remove the foam.

17. Immediately afterward, close the mold and wrap it in a blanket or towel to cool off gradually, or return it to the turned-off oven. Gradual cooling prevents a sudden change of temperature from cracking the mold.

18. You must be extremely careful when separating molds that have escape holes. Before opening them, grasp the mushroom-shaped piece of foam on top and very gently pull it up. Cut the stem with scissors.

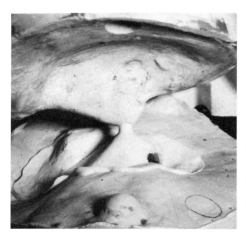

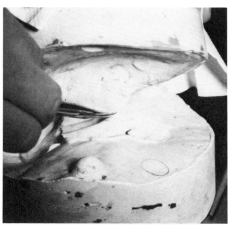

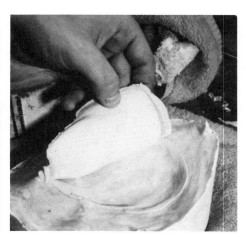

19. If there is nothing on the top of the mold, open it gently.

20. When you see the "umbilical cord," cut it off with scissors.

21. Then remove the foam.

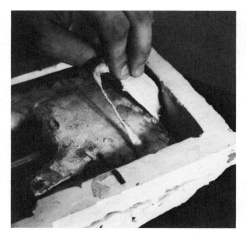

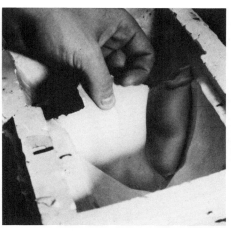

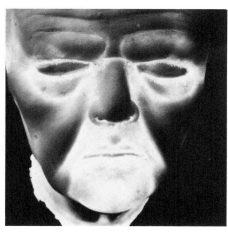

22. In the case of large molds, it is better first to remove the extra foam on top between the positive and the negative and then to cut the umbilical cord, if any.

23. Then gently remove the positive and the foam. Powder the foam right away. If it is a little damp, or if the thin edges curl under, return the mold to the oven for another half hour or so.

24. If you hold the final product in front of a light, you can see how thin the edges and other areas of the piece are. These places are easily damaged in the process of removal from the molds, so be careful.

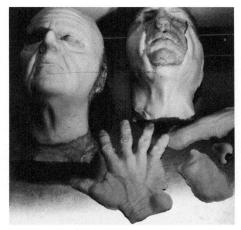

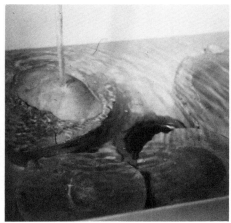

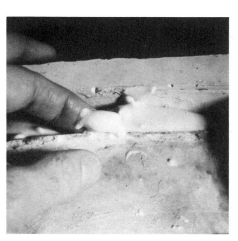

25. When all the molds for the job are out of the oven, place all the full faces over their positives. If the molds are still hot, cover them with a blanket, and allow them to cool. Place all the small pieces in a plastic bag and seal it until you are ready to use them. If they stay outside under light and in contact with the air, after a while they change color and sometimes shrink a bit.

26. These molds are good for three or four uses. If you use them twice a day, you must let them cool off in between. Later on, each time you use them, place them in a sink full of water and soak them for a minute or two. Take them out, dry them, apply the separating agent, and use them as before.

27. Now let us go back a few steps. If the foam does not jell after 15 minutes, it begins to break down and will collapse if you place the molds in the oven. The foam cannot be used, and you must clean the molds and start over.

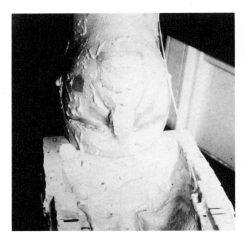

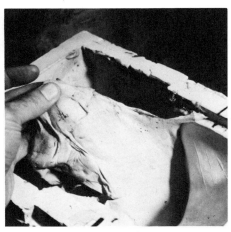

28. Cleaning the molds is a very messy job indeed. It is better to separate the molds and let them stay open to dry out for a few hours. If you are in a hurry, use a hand hair dryer to set the foam for easy removal.

29. Then you can peel each piece out of its mold very easily and start at the beginning.

Never begin the application of foam-latex pieces with one set of each appliance. Always arrive at the studio with at least three good sets of each item. One may get ruined, or the actor may need to clean his face for lunch, or heat and perspiration may damage the pieces—and you must be ready to do the makeup all over again. Needless to say, for a long production such as a film or TV show for which an actor has to wear the pieces for days or even weeks, you need a fresh appliance and backups each day.

GEORGE BAU'S FOAM

For those of you interested in working with George Bau's foam, the kit consists of:

  5 gallons of latex (as of now this is the smallest quantity you can get)
  1 pint of Sponge Curing Agent
  1 pint of Sponge Foaming Agent
  1 pint of Sponge Jelling Agent

You will find on each container the manufacturer's recommended measurements for each batch. A full batch is:

  150 grams of latex
  12 grams of curing agent
  30 grams of foaming agent
  14 grams of jelling agent

Always remember this general rule: shake all the bottles thoroughly before you begin.

1. Measure the empty mixing vessel (ours weighed 337 grams) and balance the scale.

2. Add 150 grams of weight on the other side, or move the counterweights to read 487 grams (the weight of the empty vessel plus 150 grams).

3. Pour the latex into the vessel very carefully until the scale is balanced again. If you get more than 150 grams, spoon out the excess.

4. Add 12 grams of weight to the other side of the scale, or move the counterweights to read 499 grams (vessel weight plus 150 grams of latex plus 12 grams). Add curing agent until the scale is balanced. Curing agent is a very heavy, pasty liquid, and you must pour it in almost drop by drop be-

cause you cannot remove the excess if you accidentally add too much.

5. Add 30 grams of weight, or move the counterweights to 529 grams. Add foaming agent to balance the scale. This is a light, spongy liquid; pour it very carefully.

6. Mix the three liquids in the vessel with a long spoon. The mixture is now ready to be beaten. Set the mixer at the highest speed and beat the mixture for about 6 to 10 minutes to reach a volume of 4½ or 5 inches (11½ to 12½ cm) for a soft foam. I have discovered that in the process of beating it is sometimes helpful to add eight to ten drops of ammonia. This is not in the formula. It delays the jelling of the foam and gives you more time to fill the molds. You should experiment with and without the ammonia and time the jelling under various conditions before you make your decision.

7. Set the mixer at number 3 speed and refine the foam for 3 minutes.

8. Meanwhile, measure the jelling agent. Place a 3-ounce plastic cup on the scale, balance it, and add 14 grams of weight. Pour the jelling agent into the cup to balance the scale. Then, without adding weight to the scale, add ten drops of color to the cup. Mix with a spatula or spoon.

9. When the foam has been refined for 3 minutes, add the jelling agent in the center of the vessel. With the help of a spoon or spatula at the side of the vessel, run the mixer to blend the color (see steps 10–11, page 103). After about 1 minute the foam will be evenly colored, which means that

the jelling agent is uniformly mixed with the foam. Remove the spoon or spatula and mix another 30 or 45 seconds. The foam should now be ready to pour into the molds.

Because humidity, room temperature, and other factors affect the results with this material, don't count on getting a good batch every time. For no apparent reason it might jell right in the vessel, or it might not jell at all. Jelling time can vary from 2 to 10 minutes, or even more.

As you gain experience you will change the formula. You will find it necessary to add more of one ingredient or less of another, or to beat it less or more. Whatever you do, do it carefully and write down in your log every step you take, good or bad, for future reference.

You may not need the entire 150-gram batch each time. That basic batch is good for one large or three or four small molds. You can halve the measurements for just a few small molds: 75 grams of latex, 6 grams of curing agent, 15 grams of foaming agent, 7 grams of jelling agent, and five drops of color. The beating and refining times remain the same.

In preparing the molds for this foam, apply Bau's Separating Agent sparingly over the positive and negative molds with a brush and wipe clean with your fingers. Then brush a thin coat of liquid soap over the positive and *only* over the cutting edge that frames the negative; that is, do not apply soap over the modeling itself.

CHAPTER TEN

APPLICATION OF FOAM LATEX

In this chapter we show the application of the foam-latex pieces to age our subject to forty, then fifty-five, then seventy-five.

For the first stage, age forty, we used nasolabial folds. For age fifty-five, we prepared one piece to cover the sides of the face, neck, and double chin, plus a separate chin, nose, and forehead. To complete the effect, we added a receding hairline and different hair.

For age seventy-five, we used a single piece for the face. Whether you use four pieces or just one is a matter of personal preference—the results are the same. The other factor is time—it takes longer to apply four pieces than one. I have found that there are fewer worries about thin edges, overlapping pieces, and blending when I use one piece.

You may approach the aging process in a totally different way. The details of the makeup depend on the subject's bone and muscle structure and the character he is to portray. I cannot stress enough how important continuity of muscle structure is. If you undertake a project like this, make sure you do all the modeling yourself. If you must work with others, do not cast the pieces until you have checked them all for continuity.

MATERIALS AND EQUIPMENT

Foam-latex pieces and duplicates of each piece

Spirit gum or Plastic Adhesive 355

Brushes of all sizes, straight and bent

Butterfly tweezers

Duo Surgical Adhesive

Liquid latex

Hand-held hair dryer

All shades of rubber mask grease

Red A Creme Stick

Lining colors

Stipple sponges

Foam-rubber sponge

Hair whitener

Toothbrush

Hairpieces and mustaches

Plastic bald caps

Acetone

Alcohol

Powder and powder puffs

Brush and comb

Scissors

Boxes of tissues

Base colors in Creme Sticks

Highlight and shadow colors

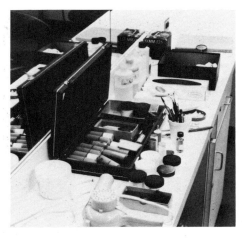

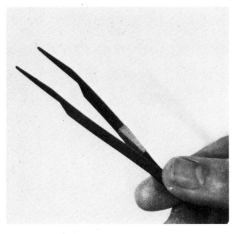

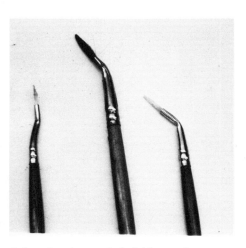

1. Prepare a list of all the items you will need a day or so ahead of time. Collect them all, and make sure they are clean and usable. Arrive at the studio at least an hour ahead of the subject. Arrange all your materials on the counter where you will work in such a way that you can reach them easily with one hand while the other is on the subject's face. Get rid of all unnecessary items; they only take up room and confuse you. Double-check everything against your master list a couple of times. Now you are ready to work.

2. For gluing foam pieces, it is essential to have a pair of butterfly tweezers. When you ease the pressure of your fingers on regular tweezers, the tips open and drop whatever they were holding. The tips of butterfly tweezers, however, remain closed when your fingers get tired and relax because of their shape and the softness of the material.

3. Bent brushes are helpful for getting under the edges of foam pieces and into hard-to-reach corners. They are regular paintbrushes; simply bend the top section slightly with your fingers or pliers.

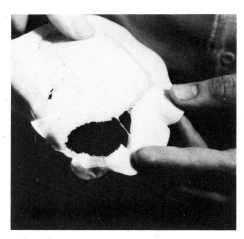

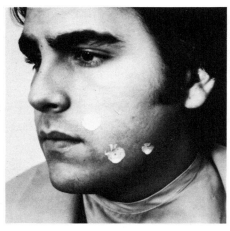

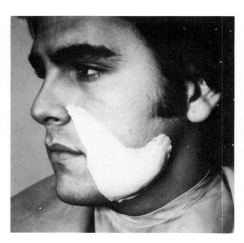

4. Remove any extraneous foam from the pieces you are going to use. Separate each piece from the overflow by gently pulling along the thin area between them. Do this carefully; if you damage these areas, the edges will be too thick.

5. Have the subject sit in a comfortable makeup chair, preferably one with an adjustable headrest, and position his head exactly the way it was when you took the life mask; otherwise the pieces will not fit properly. Make sure the subject's face is clean and free of natural oils. Apply touches of liquid latex to the subject's face where one of the appliances is to go. Move his head up and down or to the sides to get the right position.

6. Tack the piece to the face by gently pressing it down.

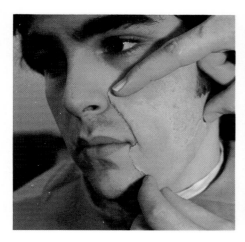

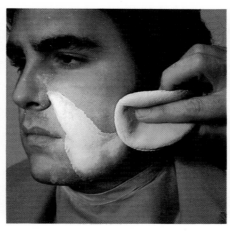

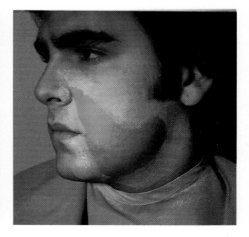

7. In this photograph the same piece is shown, already colored. In this demonstration we are going to use a white piece on one side of the face and a colored piece on the other to show the difference in the final results.

8. Powder the edges of the piece and the surrounding skin.

9. When you lift the piece, you'll find its outline. This will help you to replace the piece accurately. (After a few years of practical experience you will be able to skip steps 8 and 9.)

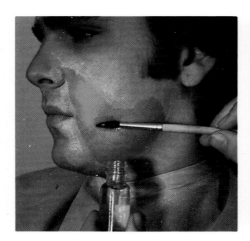

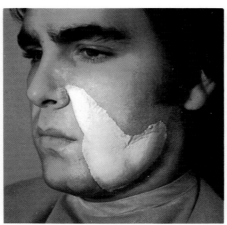

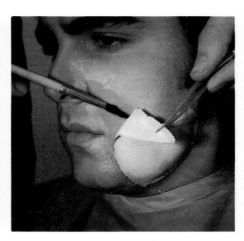

10. Brush spirit gum onto the center of the area only, using just enough to hold the piece in place. If the subject is allergic to spirit gum, you can use liquid latex, Duo Surgical Adhesive, or Plastic Adhesive 355.

11. Replace the piece gently within the powdered outlines and press to hold. Keep the spirit gum away from the thin edges of the piece.

12. Lift the upper half of the piece with tweezers and apply spirit gum to the face, starting at the edges of the last application (the center of the piece) and spreading adhesive to within about ¼ inch (6 mm) of the edge. Gently press the piece down to adhere it. Be extremely careful not to leave even the smallest area unglued—except for the edges, at this stage.

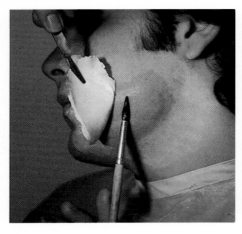

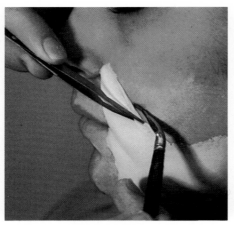

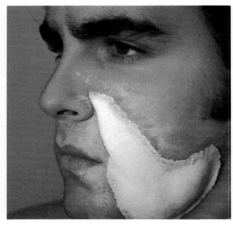

13. Lift the lower half of the piece with tweezers and apply spirit gum from where the first application ended to within ¼ inch (6 mm) of the edge. Gently press the piece down.

Why do we leave the edges unglued? Because they require the utmost care. They must blend into the skin. They should not fold under, wrinkle, stretch, or overlap. Maybe after a few years of practice you can glue the edges at the same time as the rest of the piece, but at this time I suggest that you do it step by step and very slowly.

14. Begin gluing the thin edges at the nostril. With one hand lift and bend or hold back the area you are working on with butterfly tweezers. With the other hand use a small, flat brush, ⅛ inch (3 mm) wide, straight or bent, to apply spirit gum to the skin under the piece as far out as the edge of the powdered area and perhaps a little beyond. Never apply spirit gum to the appliance itself. When the thin edges get wet and gummy with spirit gum or other adhesive material, the foam latex folds under and sticks to itself. This causes trouble.

15. Very gently lay the foam piece against the face and let it sit on the spirit gum. Make sure it falls in the right place, because it is risky to try to lift the piece and reposition it. Do not just let go of the piece; it will snap down and might not fall in the right place.

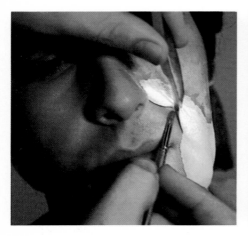

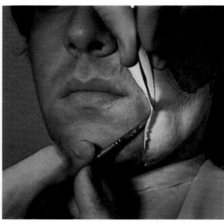

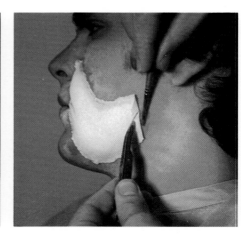

16. Now proceed to the other side of the nasolabial fold. Again lift the piece with tweezers and apply spirit gum under it. Bear in mind that the more of the piece you have glued, the harder it is to glue the next section. Take your time and handle the pieces very carefully.

17. Continue gluing the piece around the lips and chin.

18. Glue the outer section, over the jawbone.

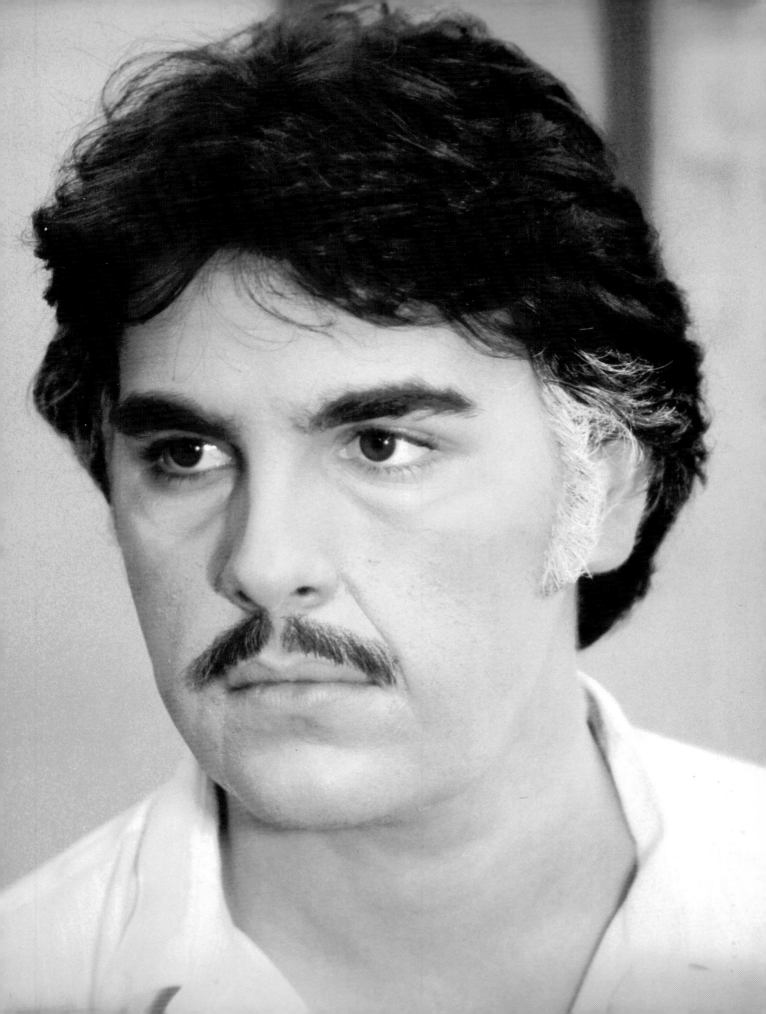

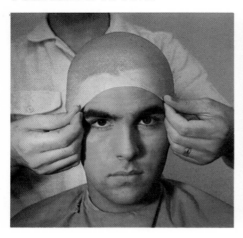

1. Because the subject will have a receding hairline and wear a wig, a bald cap is necessary. The front part of the cap will be seen, so a plastic cap of the type used for television and film is best. Comb the subject's hair down as flat as you can and put the bald cap on his head.

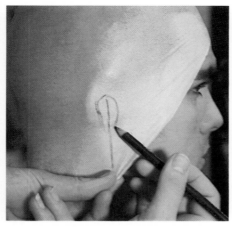

2. Mark the ears with pencil as shown.

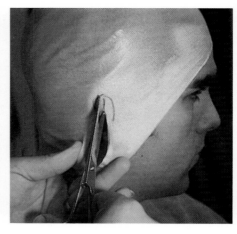

3. Cut the cap straight up to within ½ inch (13 mm) of the top of each ear.

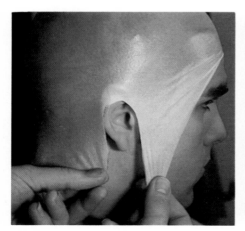

4. Then cut a semicircle. (If you cut it straight and pull the cap on both sides, it will rip easily.)

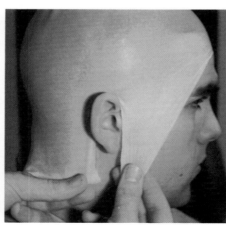

5. Pull the rear flap behind the ear and push the hair under it. Do the same with the other side. (Some makeup artists prefer to mark and cut the ear holes after the front and the back of the cap are glued.)

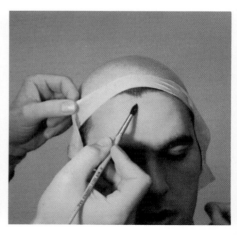

6. Lift the front of the cap and apply spirit gum to the forehead up to the hairline. Stop before you reach the temples. Let the spirit gum dry. (You can use plastic adhesive instead of spirit gum.)

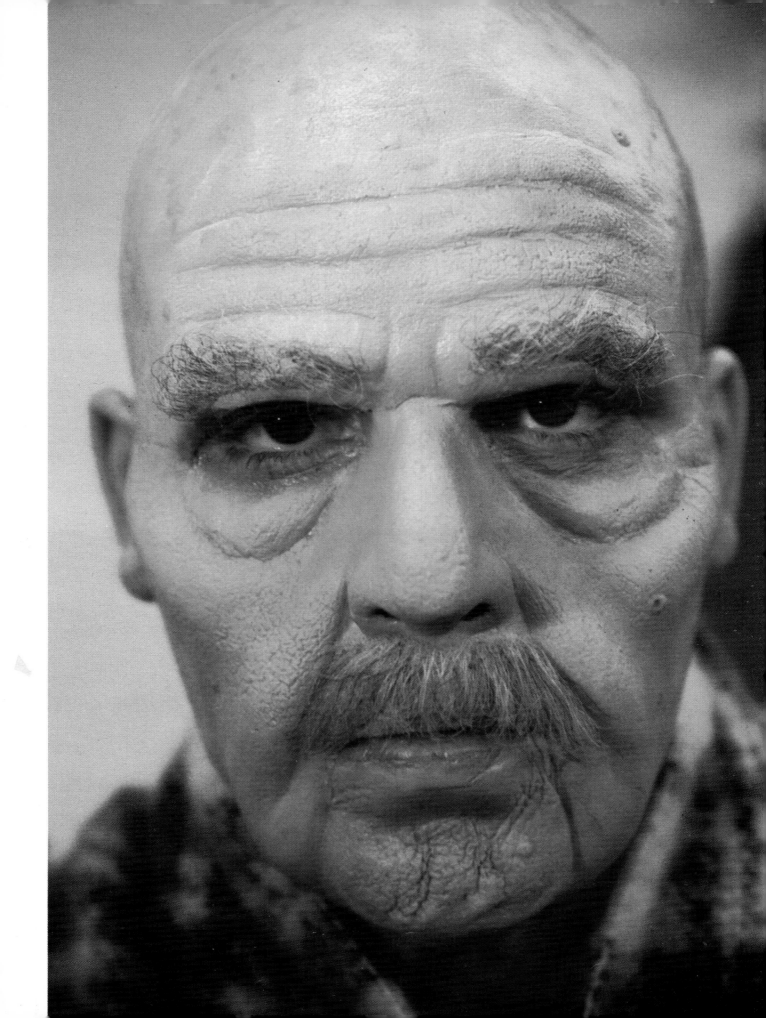

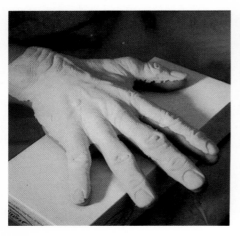

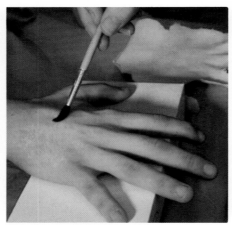

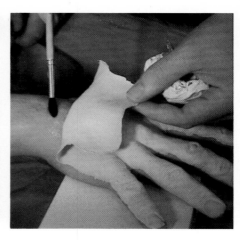

1. Place the foam-latex hand over the subject's own hand to check the fit.

2. Lift the foam piece and apply spirit gum or plastic adhesive to the back of the subject's hand.

3. Replace the foam piece and press it to hold. Lift the back section and apply spirit gum, section by section. Press the piece down to hold.

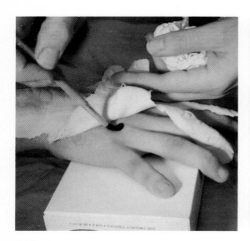

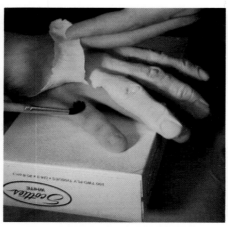

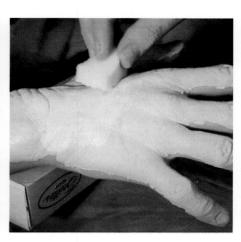

4. Do the same with the front section.

5. Then lift one finger at a time, apply spirit gum to the skin, and press the foam finger down. Be especially careful when you glue the thin edges around each finger.

6. When all the fingers are glued, apply a coat of liquid latex or Duo Surgical Adhesive all over the piece with a foam-rubber sponge. Keep the fingers spread apart. Dry with a hand-held hair dryer and powder immediately.

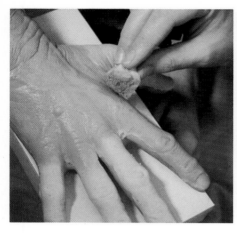

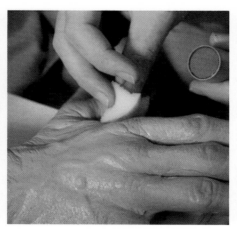

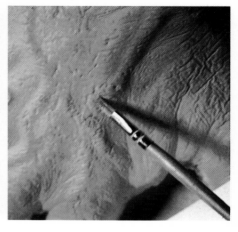

7. Select or mix the proper color in rubber mask grease and stipple it over the hand evenly, smoothly, and sparingly with a foam-rubber sponge.

8. For old-age hands add a touch of red over the knuckles. Here we used a Sunburn shade in Creme Stick.

9. Select the right shade of blue or bluish gray and color all the veins.

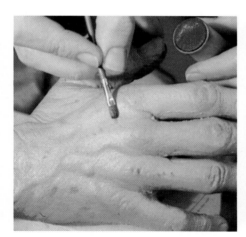

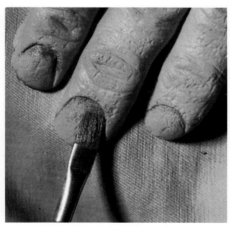

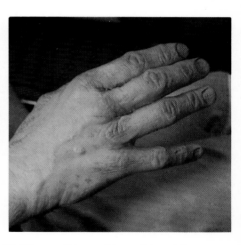

10. Add some liver spots and the other skin discolorations that old people have on their hands.

11. Because we have modeled this piece to cover the subject's fingers and fingernails, we must give the nails a touch of flesh color or maybe a yellowish tone. A little brown or black under and around the fingernails may be added.

12. The result is an old man's hand that matches the old man's face.

To apply the flat old-age hand described in Chapter Four, follow the same steps, but wrap the extended sections around each finger and overlap them wherever possible. Then follow the rest of the technique explained in this chapter.

To glue the flat piece over the surgical glove, first let the subject wear the fitting glove. Then with Plastic Adhesive 355 glue the foam over it carefully. For this the modeled hand must have fingernails as well.

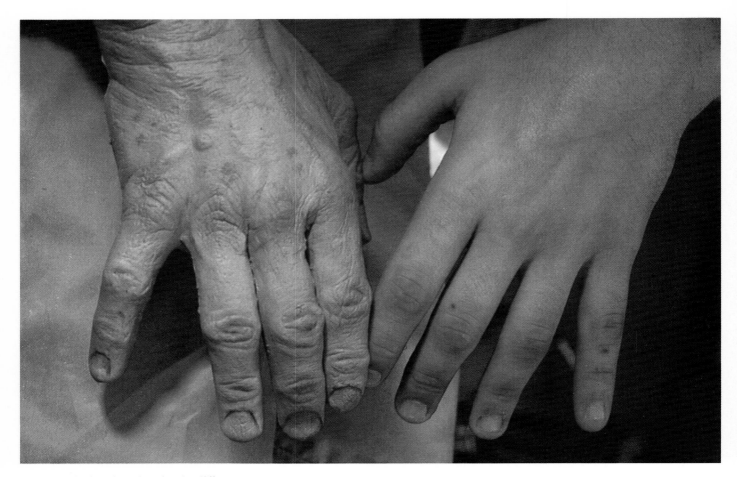

Compare the hands and notice the difference. We have done only one hand for the purpose of this book; be sure to do the other.

You must experiment, test, and use new materials that appear on the market to find the best approach to your work. What we have explained in this book is only a guide, not the final answer. There are no final answers in any art form.

To progress in your art and avoid past mistakes, and to be able to repeat the valuable work you have done in the past, carry a notebook with you on all your jobs and make notes about everything you do: colors you have used, improvisations, pieces you have discarded, what prompted you to alter your steps, and so on. This notebook can save you a great deal of trouble in the future. Each face and each job has its own unique problems, of course, but your notes will serve as an invaluable guide.

NOTES ON COLORING

I cannot emphasize enough how important the coloring is. It is an art in itself that requires understanding the colors you use, and why and where you use them. At times the coloring takes more time than the application of prosthetic pieces. The exact procedures for coloring are beyond the scope of this book. Suffice it to say, for our purposes, that you should work sparingly, delicately, and with good judgment. Don't overdo it, and never use colors merely for the sake of using them.

There is always the problem of color from the face and neck rubbing off on the subject's shirt collar, or color from the hands rubbing off on clothing. Here are two suggestions:

Instead of using rubber mask grease, mix acrylic colors with liquid latex to get the exact shade you want and stipple the color over the foam latex.

Apply one or two coats of liquid latex over the hands and face after the makeup is finished, and then dry and powder as usual.

This prevents the colors from rubbing off and gives the face a slight natural sheen. To get rid of the powdery look, rub some castor oil on top of the latex with your fingertip. Do not apply any other color over this coat of latex.

Here is a formula from Dick Smith:

"Artist's acrylic paint such as Liquitex can be made flexible enough to adhere to latex and foam latex. Add twenty to thirty drops of Monsanto's Santicizer 160 to 1 fluid ounce of any acrylic paint or medium and stir it in well.

"Plasticized acrylic will not stick to the skin, but it will stick to areas coated with latex stipple. It is useful on appliance makeup in areas where rubber mask grease is troublesome: on the neck where rubber mask grease would come off on the costume, or on any area where hair or hairpieces must be glued on.

"Acrylic gel can also be plasticized and used to cover appliance defects and bad edges."

PART FOUR:

TEETH, EARS, DUPLICATING NATURAL FEATURES, CASTING A FULL HEAD

CHAPTER ELEVEN

MAKING TEETH

At times it is necessary to change the shape and color of a character's teeth, especially if the subject is young and must portray an older person. To decide on this change, you must take into account the character's life-style, such as eating, smoking, and other habits. To be able to follow this procedure correctly on someone else, it is not a bad idea to try it on yourself first.

MATERIALS AND EQUIPMENT

Impression plates for upper and lower teeth

Nu-Gel, a powder much like the impression cream used for casting faces (each can includes measuring cups)

Temporary Bridge Resin, a finely granulated acrylic in powder form in very light to very dark tones

Liquid Temporary Bridge Resin, called Manomer, which must be mixed with Temporary Bridge Resin

Five-minute epoxy, which comes in double tubes, one containing the resin and the other the hardener

Electric tool kit, including bits for sanding, cutting, shaping (we used one called a Dremel Motor Tool Kit); you could also use sandpaper, nail files, or other substitutes

Paper cups

Narrow metal spatula

Eye dropper

Petroleum jelly

⅛-inch (3-mm) Japanese brushes

Colors

Dental stone, B-11, or Ultracal 30

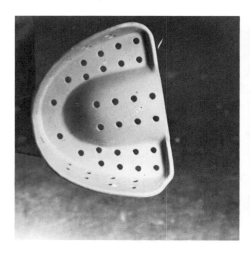

One type of impression plate is for the upper teeth.

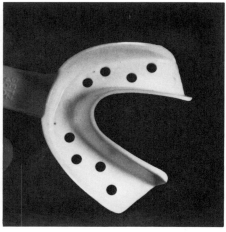

This type is for the lower teeth. The plates come in plastic or metal and in different sizes for different-size mouths.

PROCEDURE

Make this a rigid rule: *Before each application, sterilize all the items.*

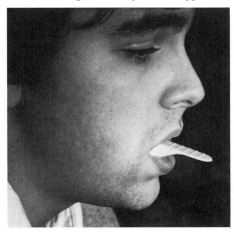

1. Try different-size impression plates in the mouth to find the right size. Put the correct one aside in a clean place.

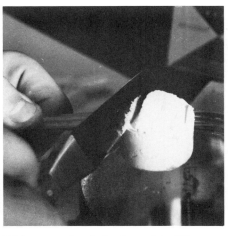

2. Measure a level plastic cupful of Nu-Gel. Pour it into a paper cup.

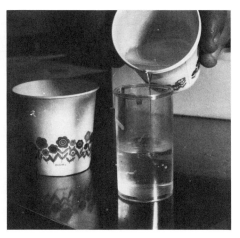

3. Measure an equal amount of water in the plastic cylindrical cup provided with Nu-Gel. Add the water to the powder.

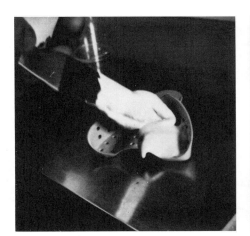

4. Mix thoroughly and fast with a spatula until you get a thick paste. Spread this paste inside the upper plate with the spatula; fill it completely. If it overflows, scrape the paste back into the plate.

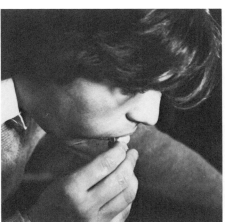

5. When the paste is about to set, open your mouth wide and put the plate inside. Close your mouth. You will feel the Nu-Gel all over your teeth and gums. Don't hurry. Don't open your mouth or move the plate. *Keep your head down*; otherwise the Nu-Gel might run down your throat, especially if it is not thick enough.

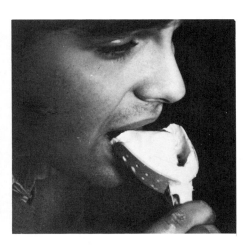

6. When the Nu-Gel is set (you can feel it or test it with your finger), loosen the plate by gently moving it from side to side. Take it out.

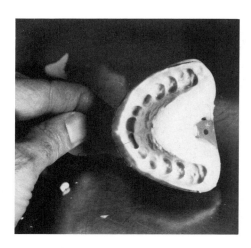

7. You will have a perfect impression of your upper teeth.

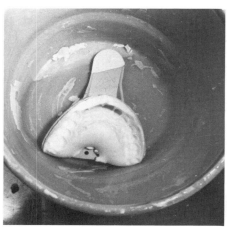

8. Submerge the plate in a bowl of cold water to prevent shrinkage while you mix the dental stone or plaster.

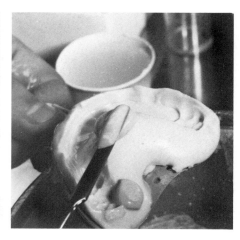

9. Mix a small amount of plaster; make it fairly thick. Take the negative out of the water, shake off the excess water, and with a small spatula or other tool insert a small amount of plaster in each tooth cavity.

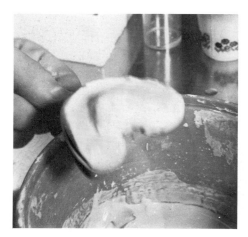

10. Shake the plate to make the plaster slide inside the cavities and to get rid of trapped air bubbles.

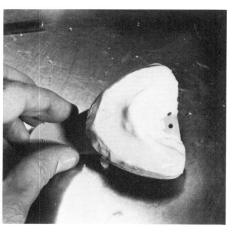

11. When all the cavities are filled, build up the plaster slightly higher than the edge of the plate and set it aside.

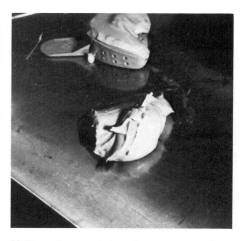

12. Pour the remaining plaster on a small area of the table (protect the table with a coat of petroleum jelly if you wish) about 1 inch (25 mm) high by 2½ inches (6 cm) wide.

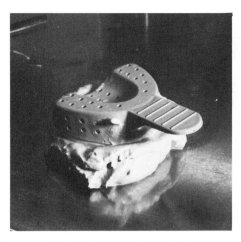

13. Pick up the plate, turn it upside down, place it on top of this lump of plaster, and gently press it down.

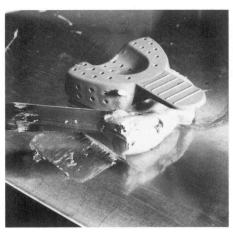

14. When the plaster is almost set, trim around it with a spatula. Let it dry completely—it will take 20 to 30 minutes.

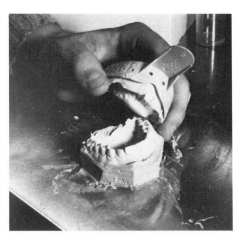

15. Remove the plate and the Nu-Gel.

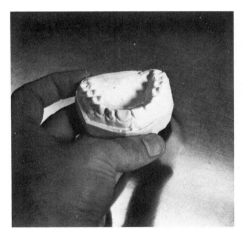

16. You have made a positive of your upper teeth.

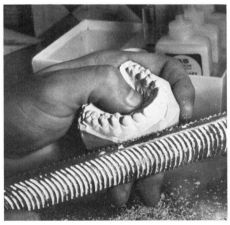

17. With a surgical knife and/or plaster rasp (shown), smooth the plaster impression to get a perfect shape.

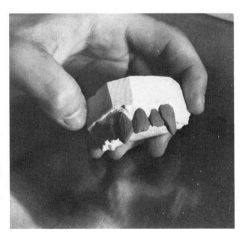

18. As for any other modeling, place a small amount of clean clay over the individual teeth you want to change and create the desired shapes with the help of modeling tools and your fingers. You can also use wax, but you must employ hot steel tools for shaping wax teeth.

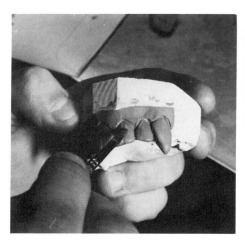

19. Continue the clay all the way up to the gum area in front.

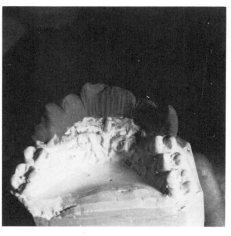

20. Continue it in the back. Make it as smooth as you can—or not, depending on what effect you have in mind.

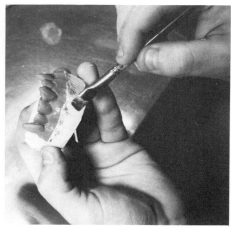

21. You must now cast the new clay or wax teeth. Apply petroleum jelly sparingly all over the modeled teeth, front and back, and over all the exposed plaster areas.

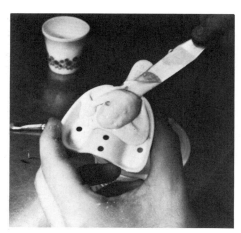

22. Follow the previous instructions (steps 2–4) for mixing another batch of Nu-Gel. Pour it as before into the empty upper plate.

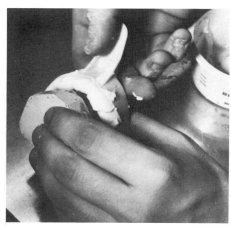

23. Before the Nu-Gel sets, press the modeled teeth into it—not too deeply or too hard, or you might damage the clay teeth.

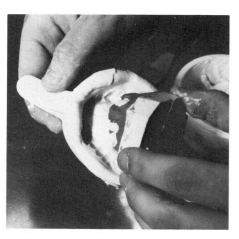

24. When the Nu-Gel is set, separate the two.

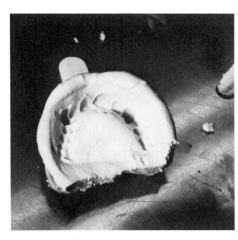

25. Some of the clay teeth may be dislodged from the positive and stay behind in the negative. Gently remove them and place the entire plate in cold water as before.

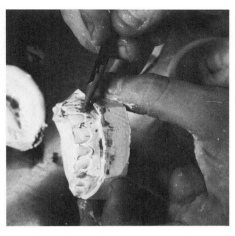

26. Clean all the clay from the positive.

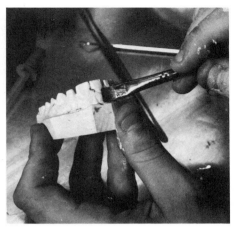

27. When it is clean, brush a coat of petroleum jelly over the plaster teeth and gums.

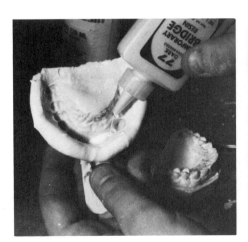

28. Remove the negative from the water and dry it. Squeeze a small amount of the proper shade of acrylic powder into the cavity of each tooth you are changing.

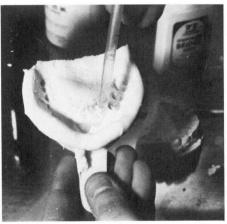

29. With an eye dropper, take up some of the liquid resin. Add it to the powder inside the mold and immediately begin to mix it with a narrow tool. You will need more powder and more liquid; add them as you go, and mix them as fast as you can.

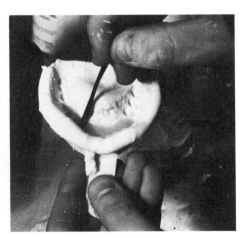

30. After all the cavities are filled, make sure there is plenty of the mixture floating around the gum; don't skimp.

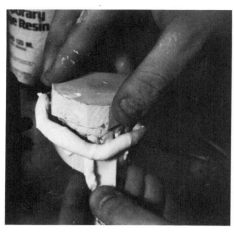

31. Place the plaster positive on top of the negative.

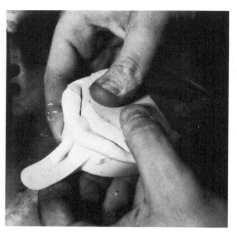

32. Press lightly until the positive is in place and the extra liquid is pushed out of the mold. Hold it for a minute; then leave it alone for 20 to 30 minutes, or until the acrylic gets hard.

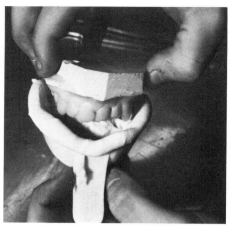

33. When it is ready, separate the pieces.

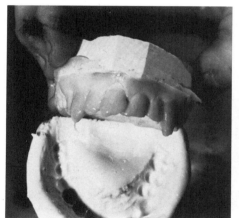

34. You have a set of new upper teeth.

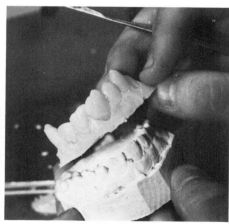

35. With a small tool pry the acrylic teeth from the mold.

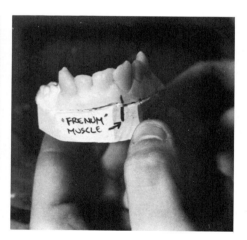

36. Place it back. Mark the center of the front gum where the frenum, the thin wall between the front gum and the upper lip, is located. (You can detect it by poking the tip of your tongue behind your upper lip.) You must cut a space on the acrylic gums so that the appliance fits on either side of this wall.

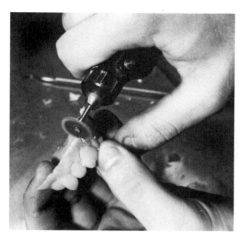

37. Use one of the bits in the electric tool kit to cut out the space.

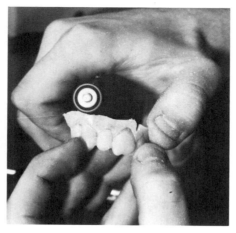

38. Use different sizes and shapes of bits to sand and smooth all the sharp edges of the acrylic teeth to make them rounded and dull. Try the appliance on a few times and see how it feels in your mouth. If you feel any discomfort, take it out, and cut it and sand it until it is comfortable.

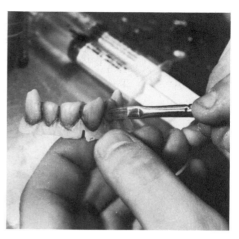

39. It is time to color the teeth with acrylics. (If you want to use wax colors instead, use Kelly's Tooth Brown Out, Black Out, and Yellow Out.) For our seventy-five-year-old man we had in mind a yellowish green, with a darker color between the teeth. First paint the dark color between the teeth.

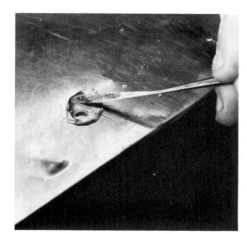

40. Squeeze a few drops of five-minute epoxy onto the table and mix the components. Add a touch of yellow for color.

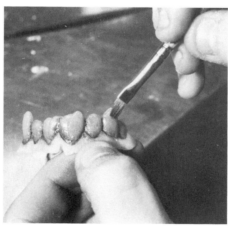

41. Brush this mixture over the teeth and let it set.

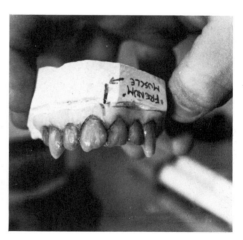

42. The new acrylic teeth are finished. For the lower teeth, follow exactly the same steps.

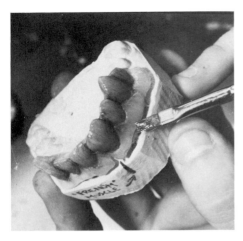

43. Add a little flesh tone to the epoxy and paint the gums with it.

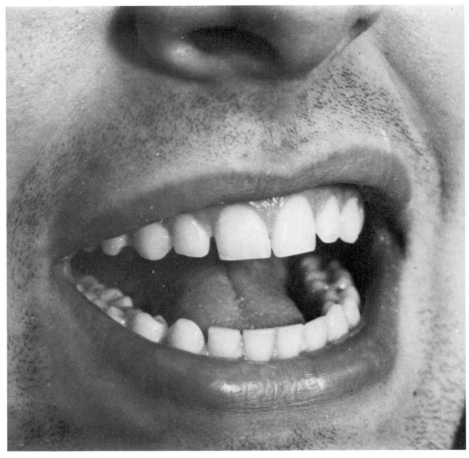

Here are the subject's natural teeth.

The new acrylic teeth have been applied.

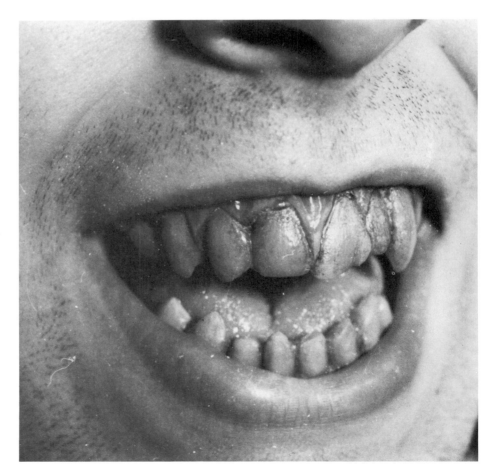

CHAPTER TWELVE
MAKING EARS

Because of the numerous undercuts, casting ears and making them different shapes with foam latex can present many technical problems, but the job is not impossible. You can make ears out of plain latex.

To begin with, you must cast the subject's ears. If you mix alginate and apply it over the ear, you will eventually get the impression, but not without creating a mess of thin areas, lumpy areas, and areas with trapped air bubbles. We have used the following technique successfully.

MATERIALS AND EQUIPMENT

Plastic container 4½ inches (11½ cm) in diameter by 3 inches (7½ cm) or 1½ inches (4 cm) high

Plastic sheets 6 by 6 inches (15 by 15 cm)

Spirit gum

Scissors

Wax

Alginate

Plastic bowls, large and small

Rubber spatula

Rubber matting

Masking tape

Surgical knife

Metal spatula

Rasp

Plaster (Ultracal 30 or B-11)

Sandpaper

Liquid latex

Hand-held hair dryer

Powder and powder puff

Cap material

Modeling clay

¾-inch (19-mm) Japanese brushes

Petroleum jelly

Foam-rubber sponge

Colors

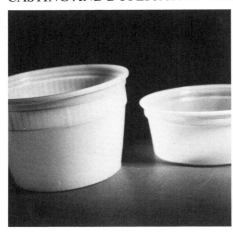

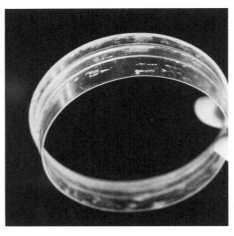

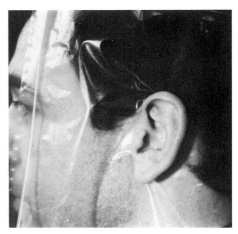

1. You can get either of these containers at a delicatessen. The large one is about 4½ inches (11½ cm) wide at the top and 3 inches (7½ cm) deep.

2. If you use the large size, cut off all but the top 1¼ inches (3 cm) with a razor blade or scissors. (Depending on the size of the subject's ears, you may need a shallower or deeper container.) If you can get the smaller size of container, 4½ inches (11½ cm) wide at the top and 1½ inches (4 cm) deep, all you have to do is cut out the bottom to make a ring.

3. Split one side of a 6-by-6-inch (15-by-15-cm) piece of plastic sheeting and fit it around one of the subject's ears.

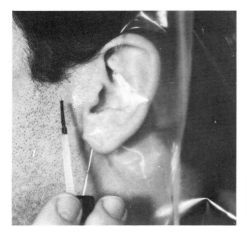

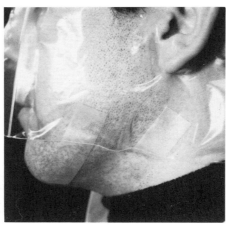

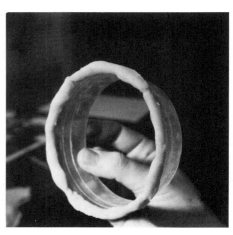

4. For a perfect casting, glue the edges of the plastic piece all around the ear with spirit gum.

5. Use Scotch or masking tape to hold the outer edges of the plastic sheet down.

6. Cover the *wider* end of the plastic ring with wax. Be sure to cover the *wider* end or you will not be able to separate the negative and positive later on.

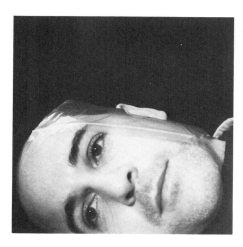

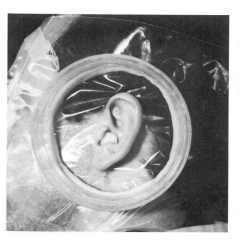

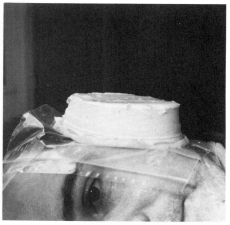

7. Ask the subject to bend his head to one side and place it on the edge of a table or over the palm of his hand. The head must remain horizontal. Insert a small piece of cotton or foam inside the ear to close the passageway.

8. Center the plastic ring over the ear, and press it down to stick to the plastic. Check all around to make sure there are no gaps under the wax. Seal any that you find with extra wax.

9. Mix a small batch of alginate to a consistency that you can pour easily. For faster setting use warm water. When it is ready, gently pour it inside the ring. Make sure the alginate goes behind, under, around, and above the ear until it is level with the top edge of the plastic container. Allow it to set.

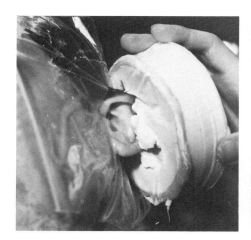

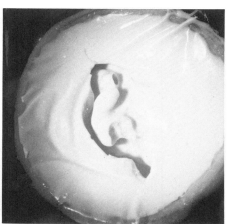

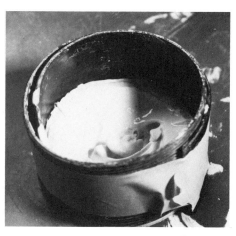

10. To remove it, separate the container from the plastic sheet, starting from front to back. (If you do it any other way you will damage the negative.)

11. You have made a perfect negative of the subject's ear. Because the alginate is thick, it will not shrink too fast, but if you have other things to do before making the positive, place the entire container in a bowl of water.

12. When you are ready to make the positive, form a wall around the container with rubber matting and secure it with masking tape. Make sure there are no gaps between the rubber wall and the edge of the container on the inside. Mix a small amount of smooth, creamy plaster. Take the air bubbles out of it.

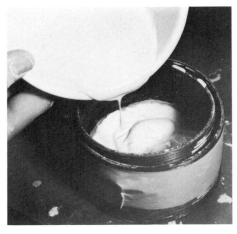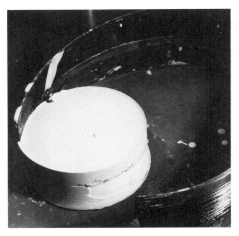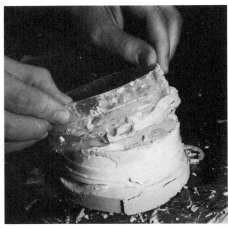

13. Pour the plaster gently inside the wall and let it fill all the crevices of the ear. You can, if necessary, squeeze the entire mold to get rid of trapped air bubbles inside the ear, because it is all soft material. Continue to pour in plaster until it is about 1 inch (25 mm) above the alginate. Let it dry.

14. Remove the rubber wall.

15. Remove the plastic container. It will slip off easily because the top side of the ring is narrower than the bottom side.

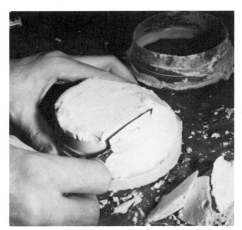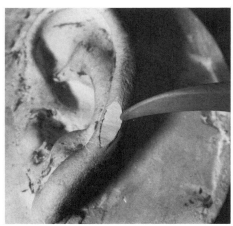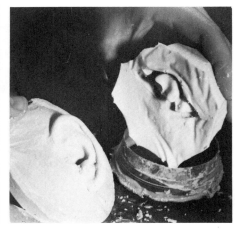

16. Cut or chip off the dried alginate with a surgical knife or spatula.

17. Be careful, however, because you can easily damage the ear, as we did here.

18. When the plaster is totally dry, you can remove the alginate from the front part of the ear toward the back. The result is a perfect positive of the subject's ear.

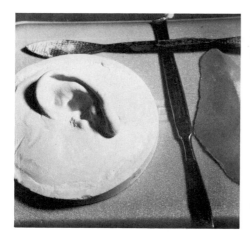

19. Use a surgical knife, rasp, or sandpaper to smooth any outer defects.

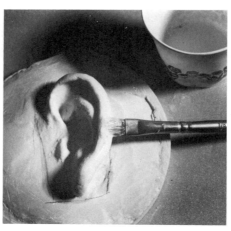

20. Brush at least ten or fifteen layers of liquid latex all over the ear, inside and out, but keep the outer edges very thin, with maybe only two or three layers.

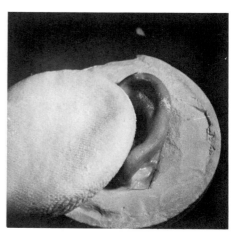

21. Dry each layer with a hand-held hair dryer and rinse the brush after each use. Let it dry totally. Powder the entire ear.

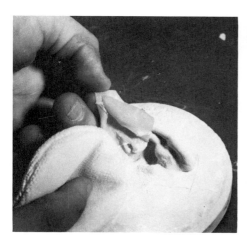

22. Gently remove the latex from the plaster. Powder it every step of the way or it will stick to itself.

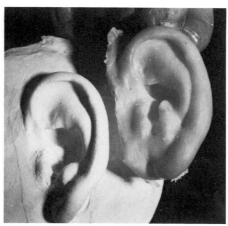

23. The result is a duplicate of the subject's ear in latex. These latex ears can be glued over the duplicate of the subject's full head (see Chapter Fourteen), provided the head was cast without the ears.

MODELING THE EAR

You may have occasion to change the shape of the subject's ear to create a specific character or to make him look very old.

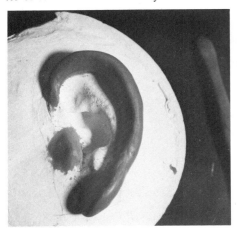

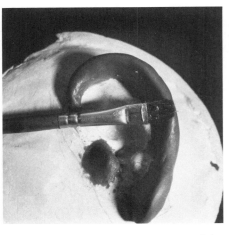

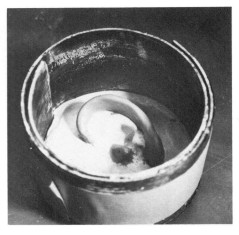

1. As for any other modeling, use clean modeling clay and model the desired shape over the plaster positive.

2. Apply a couple of layers of cap material over the clay and a coat of petroleum jelly over the plaster surrounding the modeling.

3. Place a rubber wall around the mold, mix a creamy-smooth batch of alginate, and gently pour it in. Make sure there are no trapped air bubbles, especially behind the ear.

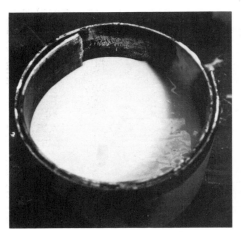

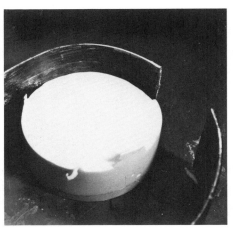

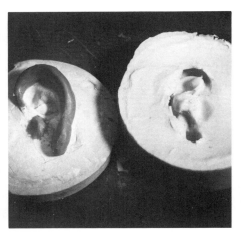

4. Fill the mold to about 1 inch (25 mm) above the highest point of the ear. Let it set.

5. When it is set, remove the rubber wall and separate the alginate from the plaster positive. Be sure to remove the negative from front to back.

6. If some of the modeling clay is left behind inside the negative, take it out with a modeling tool.

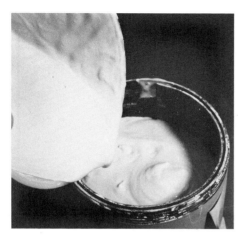

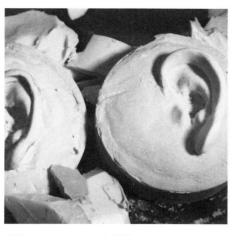

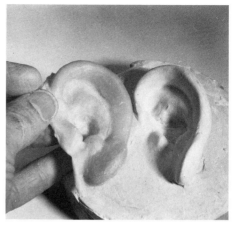

7. Put the rubber wall back around the negative and make sure there are no gaps between it and the alginate. Mix another batch of plaster and gently pour it inside the negative; squeeze the mold to get the trapped air bubbles out. When the plaster is set, remove the wall and chip off the alginate with a surgical knife or spatula. Be careful not to damage the positive.

8. The resulting ear is different in shape and size, to fit the concept of the character.

9. To duplicate this new ear in latex, follow steps 20–23 on page 151.

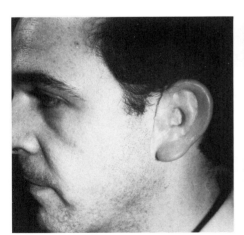

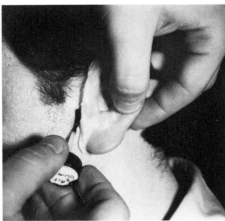

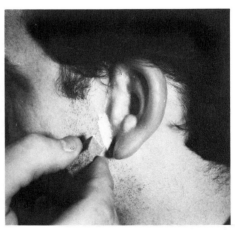

10. Place the latex ear over the subject's ear.

11. Glue the outer edges all around with spirit gum or plastic adhesive. Make sure the thin edges do not roll under.

12. Cover the entire ear with a layer of liquid latex. Dry it with a hair dryer and powder it.

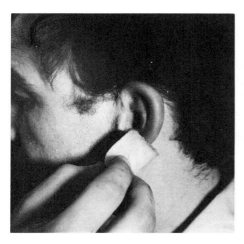

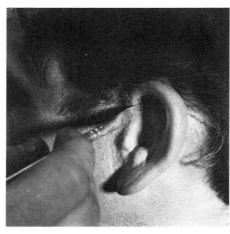

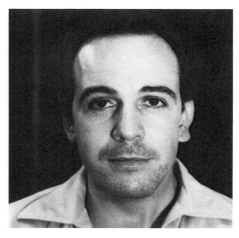

13. Color it with rubber mask grease, the same shade as the base used on the face, or acrylic colors.

14. Shade it with other colors until it looks natural.

15. The result should be a natural-looking ear.

CHAPTER THIRTEEN

DUPLICATING NATURAL FEATURES FOR STOCK USE

Instead of modeling a piece to look natural, you may simply find someone who has the kind of features you like. With the following procedure you can duplicate such pieces and add them to your stock for future use on other people. You cannot duplicate an entire face or someone else's nose, however; they will not fit other people. The only usable areas are the forehead, bags under the eyes, double chin, and nasolabial folds. Duplicating the subject's face is explained in the next chapter.

MATERIALS AND EQUIPMENT

Positive of the subject's fore-head

Modeling clay or water clay

Spatula

Rubber matting

Masking tape

Petroleum jelly

⅜-inch (10-mm) Japanese brushes

Wire cloth

Wire cutters

Pliers

Plaster (B-11 or Ultracal 30)

Electric or hand drill with ¾-inch (19-mm) router bit

Marking pen

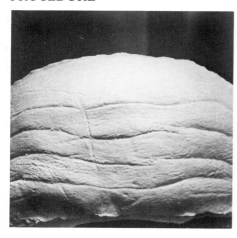

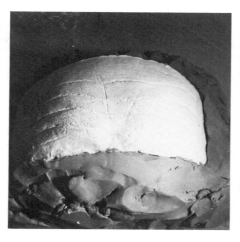

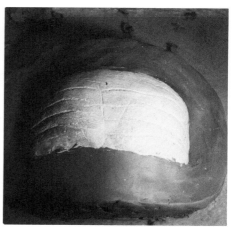

1. Suppose you like this forehead, which has been cast from someone's face. To make a similar positive to be used on someone else, follow steps 1–6 on pages 61–62.

2. After you have made the positive, place it on the table and with modeling clay or water clay build around it an extension about 1½ inches (4 cm) wide. The height of the extension must correspond to the height of the piece. Here the center is higher than the two sides.

3. Smooth the clay as best you can and trim the edges straight with a spatula.

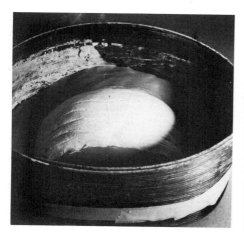

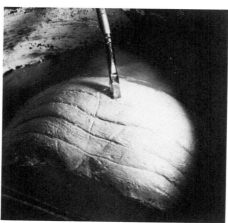

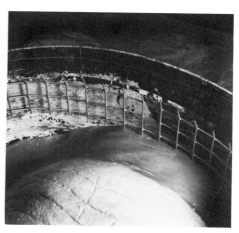

4. Form a wall around the piece with rubber matting. Make it as tight as you can and secure it with masking tape. Be sure that the clay touches the rubber wall on the inside.

5. Brush petroleum jelly over the forehead. Cover the wrinkles and lines well but do not fill them.

6. Because this mold will be used as a stock piece and baked more than once, it is a good idea to use wire reinforcement (see Chapter Two).

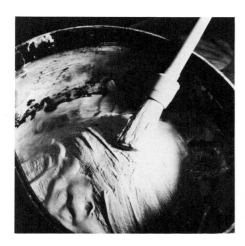

7. Mix a smooth batch of plaster and take the air bubbles out of it by hitting the bowl on the table. Brush a layer of plaster inside the mold. While the first layer sets, rinse the brush in clean water. Mix another batch and add the second layer. Let it set while you mix a larger batch in a larger bowl.

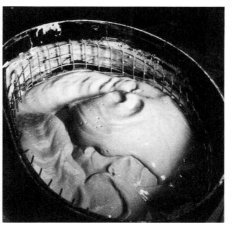

8. When that batch is ready, gently pour the plaster inside the mold from one end and let it spread by itself. After the plaster is about 1 inch (25 mm) deep, insert the wire reinforcement and pour in the rest of the plaster.

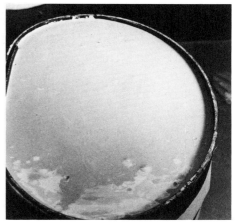

9. Mix more plaster and pour it in to cover the wire reinforcement. Let it dry thoroughly.

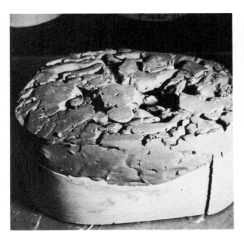

10. Remove the rubber wall and turn the mold upside down.

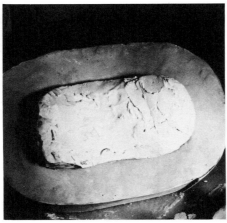

11. Remove all the clay.

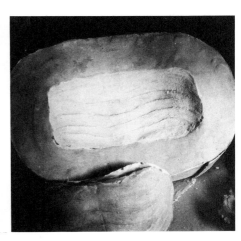

12. Gently snap off the positive and you have a perfect negative of the forehead. To be able to duplicate this forehead in foam latex you must have a positive as well.

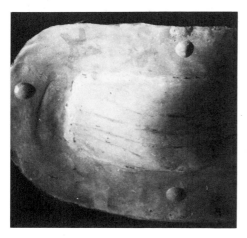

13. Before doing anything else, drill the keys (see Chapter Two).

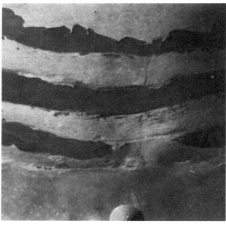

14. Spread a thin layer of clean clay inside the negative—but only over the forehead.

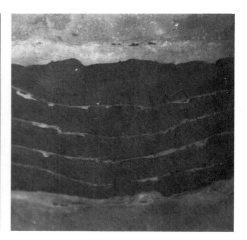

15. First fill the space between the lines of the forehead to ensure that you do not pile up a heavy layer.

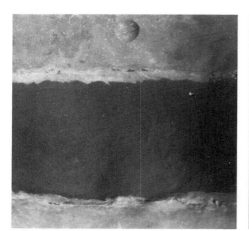

16. Go over the lines with a thin layer of clay and smooth the whole area. Keep the clay away from the edges of the forehead by about ¼ inch (6 mm) all around to ensure that you will get thin edges in the foam.

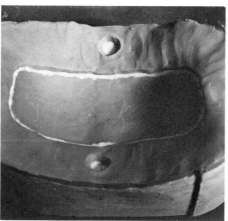

17. As for any other mold, build the cutting edge and overflow around the center section and around the keys.

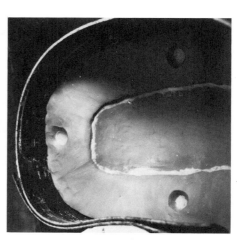

18. Wrap a rubber wall around the mold and secure it with masking tape.

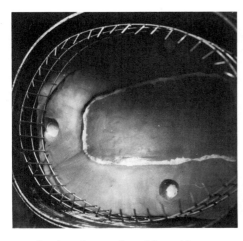

19. Like the other section, this mold requires wire reinforcement.

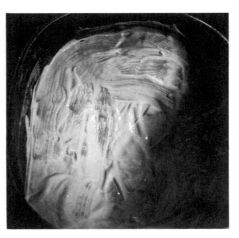

20. Mix a small amount of plaster, get the air bubbles out of it, and brush on the first couple of layers.

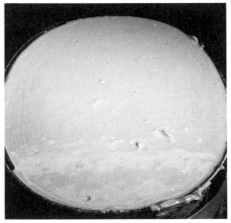

21. While these layers are setting, mix a larger batch of plaster, pour about 1 inch (25 mm) of it inside the mold, and insert the wire ring. Pour in the rest of the plaster to cover the wire ring and let it dry.

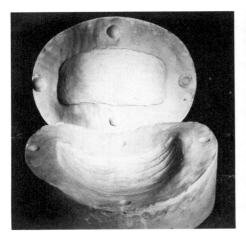

22. When the plaster is totally dry, remove the rubber wall and separate the molds. Remove the clay, clean the mold, and you have a positive and a negative.

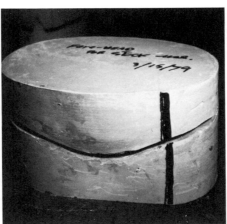

23. Mark the top and bottom to ensure proper fit, put the subject's name and date on it, and when you need it make a foam-latex piece with it. After it has been in and out of the oven a few times, soak the mold in water for a couple of minutes before use, dry it, and use it again.

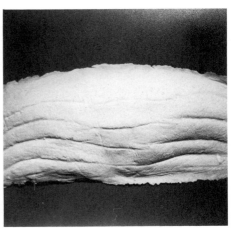

24. This is the result: a piece of foam latex with natural textures and perfect wrinkles ready to be used. As you can see, it is an exact duplicate of the original piece.

CHAPTER FOURTEEN

CASTING A FULL HEAD

Let us say you have been asked to duplicate an actor's full face or his entire head in latex or plaster for display, or for use in film or television. Modeling such a look-alike face or head, unless you are an excellent sculptor, is not an easy task. But it is not necessary, because you can cast the subject's entire head and duplicate it as often as you need it in latex or plaster.

Chapter One of this book explains step by step how to cast a face. Here we explain how to cast an entire head.

MATERIALS AND EQUIPMENT

The only materials you need in addition to those listed in Chapter One are the following:

Extra alginate, water, and plaster bandages

Molding wax

Acetone

Celastic

Five-minute epoxy

Someone to help you

CASTING THE WHOLE HEAD

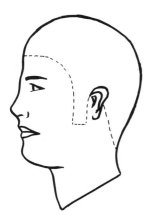

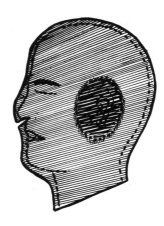

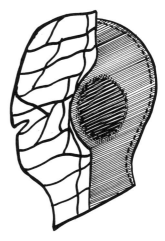

1. Follow the procedure for fitting the bald cap and preparing the subject as described in Chapter One, steps 1–9, pages 14–15. Insert a small piece of cotton, foam, or wax in the ear to close the passageway. Also place some wax behind the ears to take care of the undercuts. A touch of petroleum jelly all over the ears, inside and out, will help, too.

2. Mix the alginate and cover the entire head with it, except for the nostrils. Make the alginate at least ¼ inch (6 mm) thick all around, except an area of about 4 by 4 inches (10 by 10 cm) around the ears. Apply an extra-thick layer of alginate over the ears and taper it gradually toward the edges. It is a good idea to have someone to help you as you do the front of the face. Your co-worker can do the back and connect it to the front in the center.

3. When the alginate is set, cover the front of the face with a few layers of plaster bandages. Pass them in a straight line over the head, and curve them around the thick area of the ears and down to the neck. The thickness of the plaster bandages at the center line must be at least ½ inch (13 mm), and it must be very smooth, like a short wall.

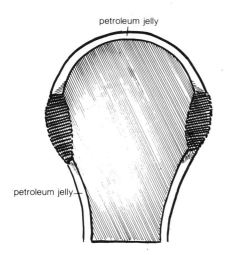

petroleum jelly

petroleum jelly

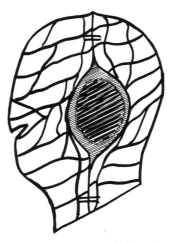

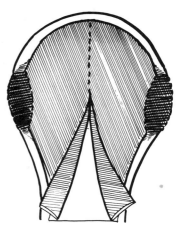

4. Brush petroleum jelly over this short wall all around.

5. Apply the same amount of plaster bandages to the back half of the head, connecting them all around to the bandages in front except at the ears. Curve the plaster bandage around the thick alginate and down to the neck. Before removing the plaster bandages, mark both halves with a single or double line, above the ears and at the neck. This will help you to put the two halves together accurately later on.

6. When the plaster is dry, gently remove the back half and with surgical scissors or a spatula split the alginate all the way to the top of the head. Carefully remove the entire life mask. You will have some difficulty releasing the ears, but because the alginate is thick there you can place your fingers under it and force the ear out without damage. Nevertheless, be extremely careful. Do not remove the front shell, if you can help it, because no matter how careful you are it is not easy to replace the alginate in the same place in the shell.

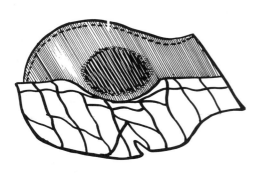

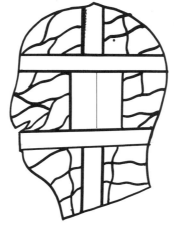

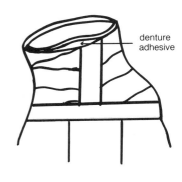

denture
adhesive

7. Before replacing the back shell, close the nostrils with wax, modeling clay, or alginate (see Chapter One, steps 27–28, page 19). Hold the entire head horizontally on your lap and glue the back seam together, very carefully, with Krazy Glue. Then replace the back shell. Make sure the pen marks meet.

8. By this time your co-worker should have prepared strips of Celastic. Soak each strip in acetone, place it over the seam, and press to shape and hold it. Cover the exposed alginate (the ear areas) with Celastic. For extra protection, add two bands of Celastic across the two halves, all around. Allow everything to dry. All this has to be done quickly to keep the alginate from drying out and shrinking. The shrinkage will be minimal if you apply the alginate thickly. It also helps to put together the split at the back of the head.

9. If the alginate separates from the outer shell at the neck, secure it with a little denture adhesive squeezed between the outer and inner sections.

To make the positive, you can brush the plaster inside the negative, but this is not easy because of its shape. You can also make a batch of plaster, pour it into the negative, and move it around until every part is covered. Continue until the plaster is ½ inch (13 mm) thick. Let it dry; then cut the Celastic guards with a razor blade, separate the two halves, and remove the alginate.

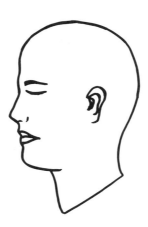

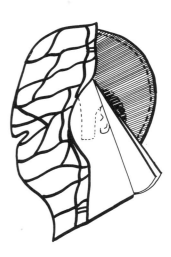

10. The result is a positive of the subject's head in plaster.

If you prefer to make a two-piece mold, follow the procedure through step 5, then skip to step 11.

11. Use a spatula to cut the alginate right where the front shell ends. Take the back piece off and place it in its own shell (be careful when releasing the ears), and place wet paper towels inside to keep it from shrinking. Remove the front half. Fill the nostrils. Now you have two half shells. Fill them individually with plaster about ½ inch (13 mm) thick. Because you are going to glue the two halves together, make the edges of the molds as smooth and clean as you can. When dry, remove the plaster bandages and alginate. Glue the two halves together with five-minute epoxy. You must fill any openings at the seam with extra plaster. Sand it smooth to give the appearance of having no seam at all.

CASTING A NEGATIVE

Now you are ready to make the negative of the head for duplication in either plaster or latex. We have chosen to do the demonstration with a clay mask that has many undercuts and crevices. We shall use PMC-724, made by Smooth-on, Inc., to make a rubber negative mold. You can follow the same steps if you are using the plaster positive instead of clay.

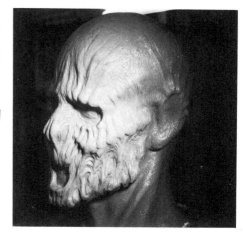

1. This is the clay mask we are going to use.

▰▰▰▰▰MATERIALS AND EQUIPMENT▰▰▰

PMC-724 consisting of:

> One bottle of Part A, the catalyst (dark brown)
>
> One gallon of Part B, the base, a creamy white latex
>
> One bottle of Part D, the harderner (clear)
>
> One container of Sonite seal release (wax)

Liquid green soap

Cab-o-Sil

Cap material

Acetone

One or two synthetic brushes 1 inch (25 mm) wide

Four disposable half-pound plastic containers

Tongue depressors

Scale

Oven

Latex

Muslin towels

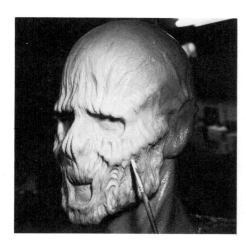

2. Apply at least three coats of cap material all over the clay model. Allow each layer to dry before you apply the next. (Clean the brush in acetone.)

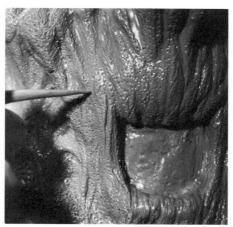

3. When the cap material is dry, you can add additional textures to the modeling, but not if you are casting a plaster piece.

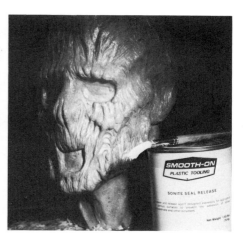

4. Paint a layer of Sonite seal release over the entire head.

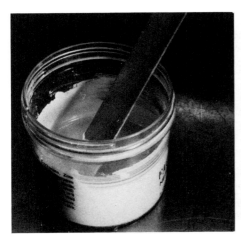

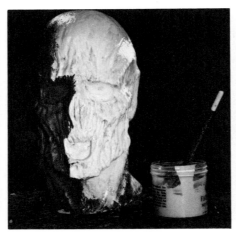

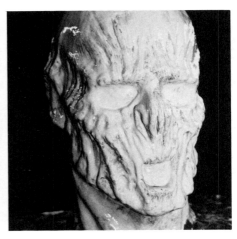

5. Measure 12 grams of Part A, 100 grams of Part B, and 2 tablespoons of Cab-O-Sil. (We use Cab-O-Sil as the thickener because material thickened with Part D does not always set on Plastilina.) Pour them into a disposable plastic container or large waxed-paper cups and mix thoroughly with a wooden tongue depressor. Set this mixture aside and measure the same amounts again into another container. Put it aside also.

6. To protect your brush, dip it in green liquid soap and rub off the excess. Brush a coat of the mixture in the first container all over the clay model. The material is not runny, like latex, so it is very easy to trap air bubbles under it. You must be very careful not to allow this to happen. There is no need to rush, because the material does not set or dry immediately.

7. When you have used up the mixture in the first container, apply the second mixture as the second layer. These two containers might be enough for two full coats. If not, you can mix more. The amounts given here can be changed. You can double the quantities or cut them in half, depending on the size of the piece you are casting.

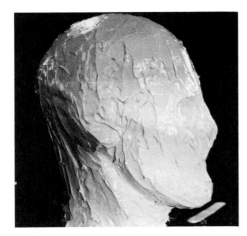

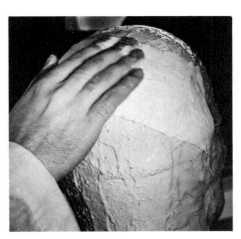

8. Mix 100 grams of Part B and 2 grams of Part D thoroughly. Then add 12 grams of Part A. (You may change the quantities as long as the proportions are the same.) The mixture soon becomes very thick and hard to mix, but you must mix all three as well as you can. Pour the mixture into another container to make sure no unmixed Part B is in the bottom or sides. Put this mixture aside and prepare another container of it. Begin applying the mixture in the first container with a wooden or regular spatula or a tongue depressor. Be careful not to trap any air. The thickness after both batches are applied should be about ¼ inch (6 mm).

We have used, after the first two coats, 1,000 grams of Part B to 20 grams of Part D and 120 grams of Part A.

The first time we did this, we left the head in the lab overnight to cure. The next day, however, it was just as wet—over the weekend the temperature of the lab had fallen below 60° F. (16° C.). We managed to remove all the material without damaging the modeling; the first two layers were better cured and made the cleaning job easier. The separation process took off a great part of the cap material and wax. To clean the surface of the clay model, we brushed methylene chloride over it. Then we repeated steps 1–8, but this time we placed the cast head in a warmer room, about 70° F. (21° C.). It was cured the next day, but even then the surface remained slightly tacky. It must be completely dry before you can continue.

9. Because of the unusual undercuts, we decided to use a three-piece shell. We used four layers of plaster bandages, instead of the usual one, to cover the back of the head.

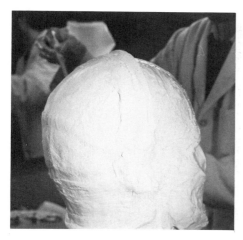

10. We also created a ¼-inch (6-mm) wall with strips of plaster bandage passed over the ears.

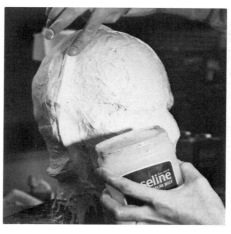

11. When this section was dry, we saturated the wall with petroleum jelly and divided the face into two halves.

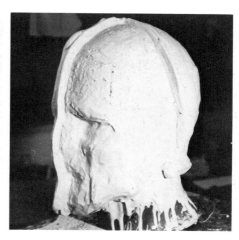

12. We applied the same thickness of plaster bandages first on one side of the face, passing over the center of the nose, upper lip, and chin, to create the same ¼-inch (6-mm) wall. When it was dry, as before, we applied petroleum jelly to the center wall.

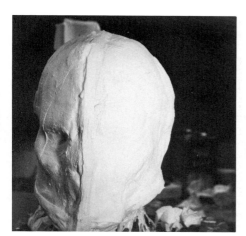

13. We finished the third section the same way.

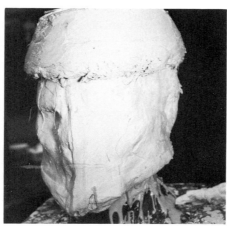

14. In order to get this cone-shaped mold straight when it is upside down, mark the top, saturate it with petroleum jelly, and build a cap with sisal fibers (you can also use loosely woven burlap) soaked in plaster. Then smooth the top and let it dry.

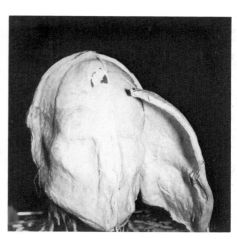

15. First remove the cap; then separate the three sections.

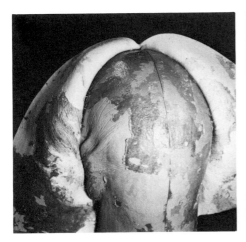

16. With a razor blade, cut the rubber mold from the top of the head down to the neck and gently peel it off.

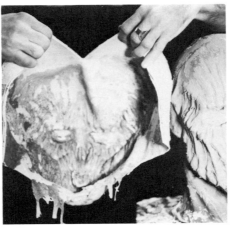

17. Some of the wax and cap material will be removed in the process and stick to the rubber mold. Rub the cap material under running tap water and in no time it will come clean.

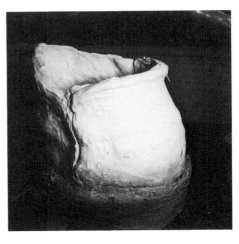

18. Place the rubber mold inside its three shells. Make sure everything fits accurately, and then place it inside the cap or base.

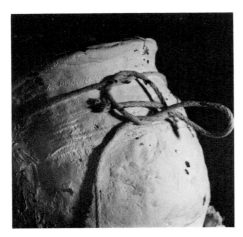

19. To hold the three-piece shell together, wrap masking tape or rope around it.

The mold is now ready to be used to make a duplicate in plaster, latex, or any other material you choose, without using any separating agent. It is a good idea to run controlled tests before using a particular material; otherwise you could ruin the mold.

For a plaster head, brush the plaster inside the mold to the thickness you want, as before. When it is totally dry, remove the shells, peel off the rubber mold, and you will have a positive of the subject's head.

We needed latex duplicates. Instead of regular latex, we used pure, thick latex from Polymer Chemical Company. It is very thick in the drum, but you can thin it out by adding some regular latex to get the consistency you need. The thicker it is, the fewer layers you will use, but at the same time it takes longer for each layer to dry.) Keep track of how many layers you use so that you can make all the duplicates the same thickness. We decided that the first two layers should be thin, but not runny, to get in and around all the crevices and undercuts, and the other five coats thicker. After adding each layer, we placed the mold in the oven at a low temperature (60° F. or 16° C.). This kept the mold warm at all times, which in turn aided the layers to dry faster. After the fifth layer, we added a couple of layers of muslin towels, cut into sections and saturated with latex, to the inside of the mold. We left the mold in the oven for a couple of hours to cure.

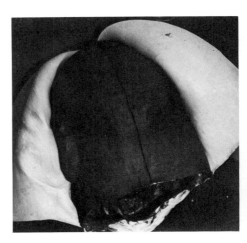

20. Remove the mold when it is dry. Separate the shells and peel off the rubber head.

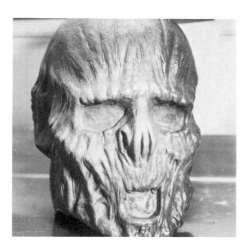

21. The result is a duplicate of the original mold in latex.

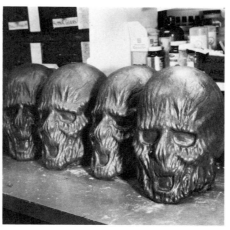

22. You can repeat the process as many times as you want. You will find, however, that after a few times—in our case twelve—the ammonia in the latex reacts to the heat of the oven and shrinks the rubber mold. The seam in the back will not meet as it did at first.

To color this mask, you can mix acrylic color with latex to the shade you need and stipple it over the latex mask. This coloring is permanent. Or you can, as we have done, add the basic coloring to the latex before it is brushed in the mold. Actually, if you color the latex for the first two layers, the rest can be used without color. You will still need to add highlights and shading to make the mask interesting and natural.

PMC-724 can be used to make other types of molds if you need to duplicate them. It lasts longer than plaster, and it is easier to use for pieces with many undercuts. If you use it over a plaster mold, you must apply a few layers of cap material first, and then go over it with wax and follow the rest of the steps.

Depending on how critical the work is, you can make a two-piece mold of the original positive with Ultrocal 30 instead of plaster bandages and make as many plaster positives and as many individual parts of the subject's face as you need.

1. Divide the head into two sections: the front, including the ears, and the back. Build a 4-inch (10-cm)-high wall of water clay between the two sections, and with a modeling tool dig out two kinds of keys: short cylinder shapes near the line where the clay touches the head, and round keys near the top of the wall. Then follow steps 15 to 23, but be especially careful about deep undercuts; fill them with PMC-724. Make the thickness of the entire surface about ¼ inch (6 mm) and of the outer edge about 1 inch (25 mm). Above all, *do not* brush the PMC-724 on the entire wall, but only halfway up, covering the cylindrical keys. Let it dry overnight, and then use a backing of Ultrocal 30 about 1 inch (25 mm) thick with good burlap reinforcement all over. When it is totally dry, remove the clay wall and repeat steps 15 to 23 (use petroleum jelly on the plaster wall) and add the back piece.

2. Before separating the two halves, drill a few holes at the center wall, passing through both sections, and use nuts and bolts to secure it. Remove the nuts and bolts, separate the two halves, peel the PMC, and take the positive out. Put the entire piece back together with all the keys fitting, tighten the nuts and bolts—and the mold is ready.

GALLERY

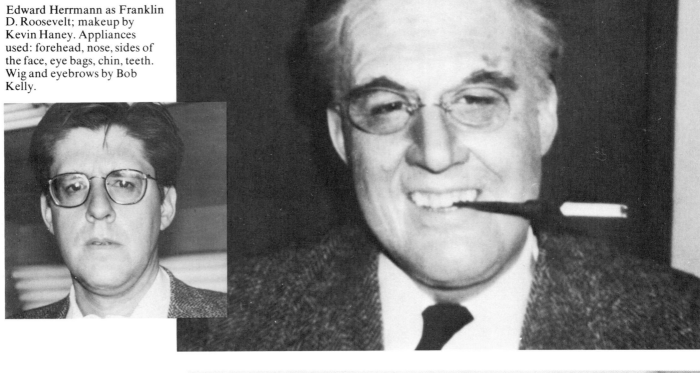

Edward Herrmann as Franklin D. Roosevelt; makeup by Kevin Haney. Appliances used: forehead, nose, sides of the face, eye bags, chin, teeth. Wig and eyebrows by Bob Kelly.

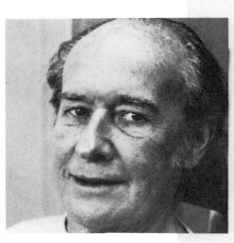

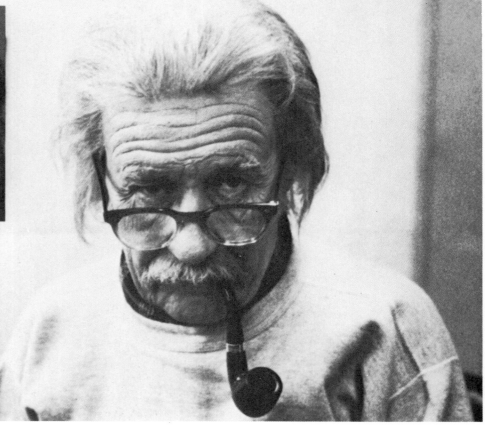

George Vascovec (this page) and Robert Blossom (opposite) as Albert Einstein. Kevin Haney made up Mr. Blossom with appliances for brows, nose, sides of the face and jowls combined, chin, and earlobes. Lee Baygan used only a forehead and nose on George Vascovec, aging the rest of his face and neck with old age stipple. Both result in a good likeness. Wigs and mustaches for both by Bob Kelly.

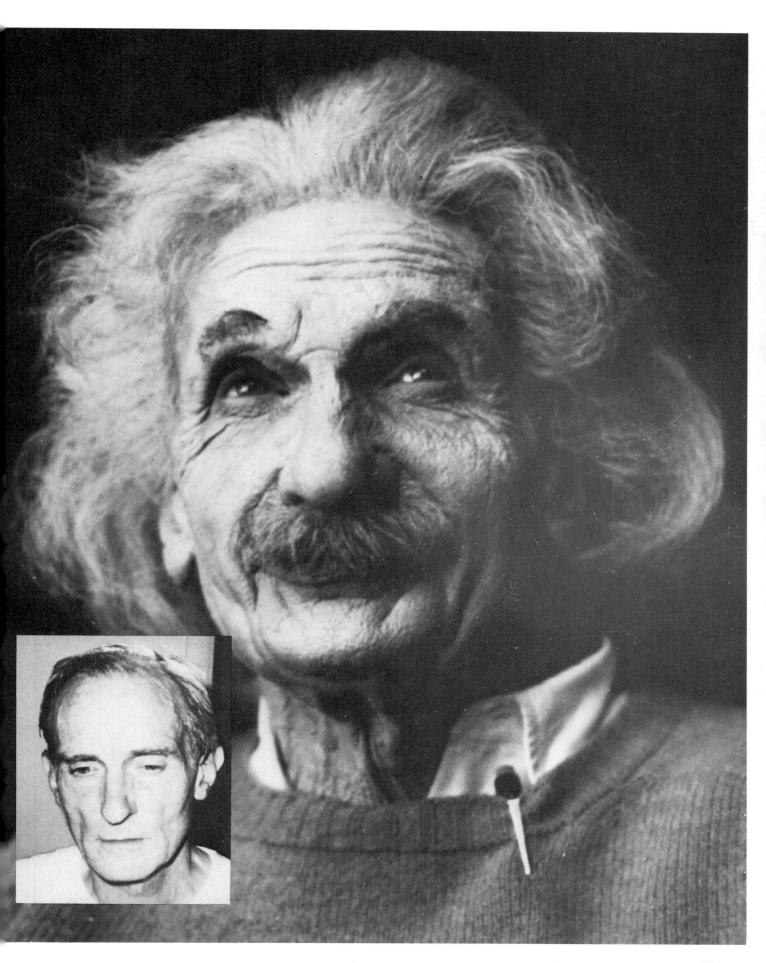

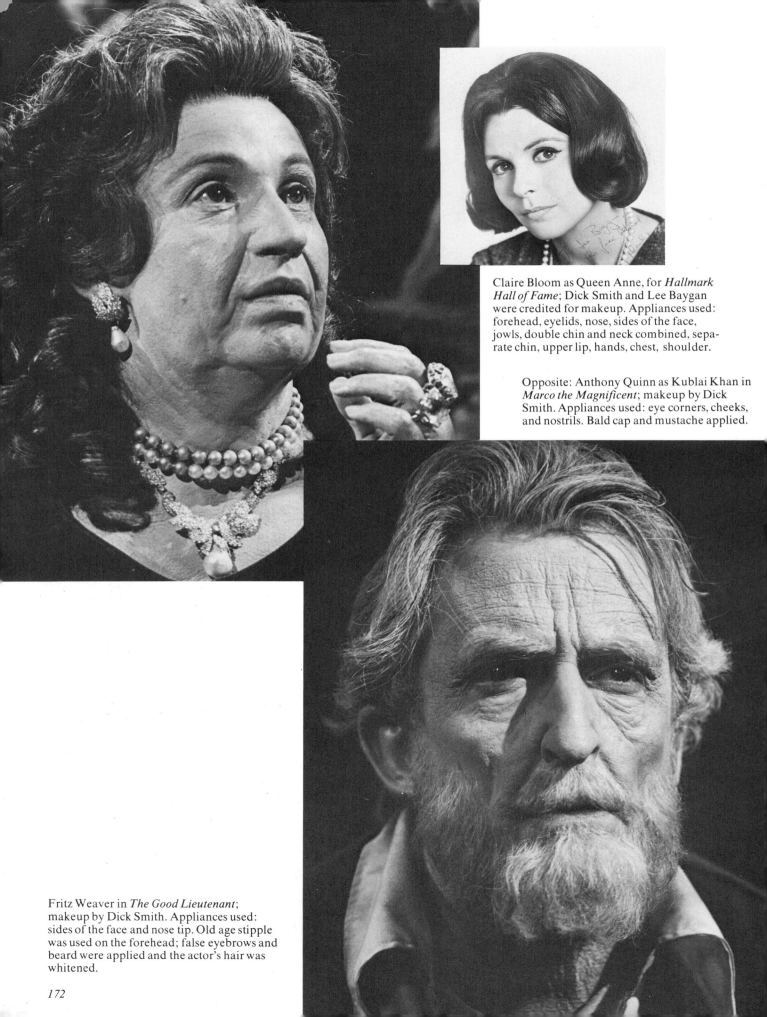

Claire Bloom as Queen Anne, for *Hallmark Hall of Fame*; Dick Smith and Lee Baygan were credited for makeup. Appliances used: forehead, eyelids, nose, sides of the face, jowls, double chin and neck combined, separate chin, upper lip, hands, chest, shoulder.

Opposite: Anthony Quinn as Kublai Khan in *Marco the Magnificent*; makeup by Dick Smith. Appliances used: eye corners, cheeks, and nostrils. Bald cap and mustache applied.

Fritz Weaver in *The Good Lieutenant*; makeup by Dick Smith. Appliances used: sides of the face and nose tip. Old age stipple was used on the forehead; false eyebrows and beard were applied and the actor's hair was whitened.

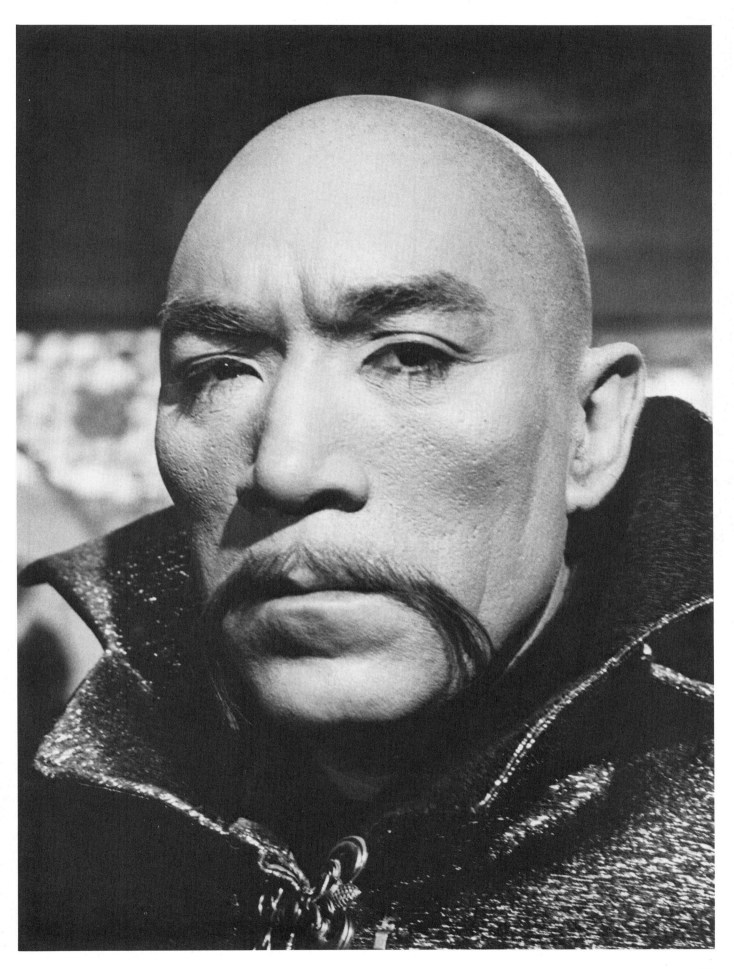

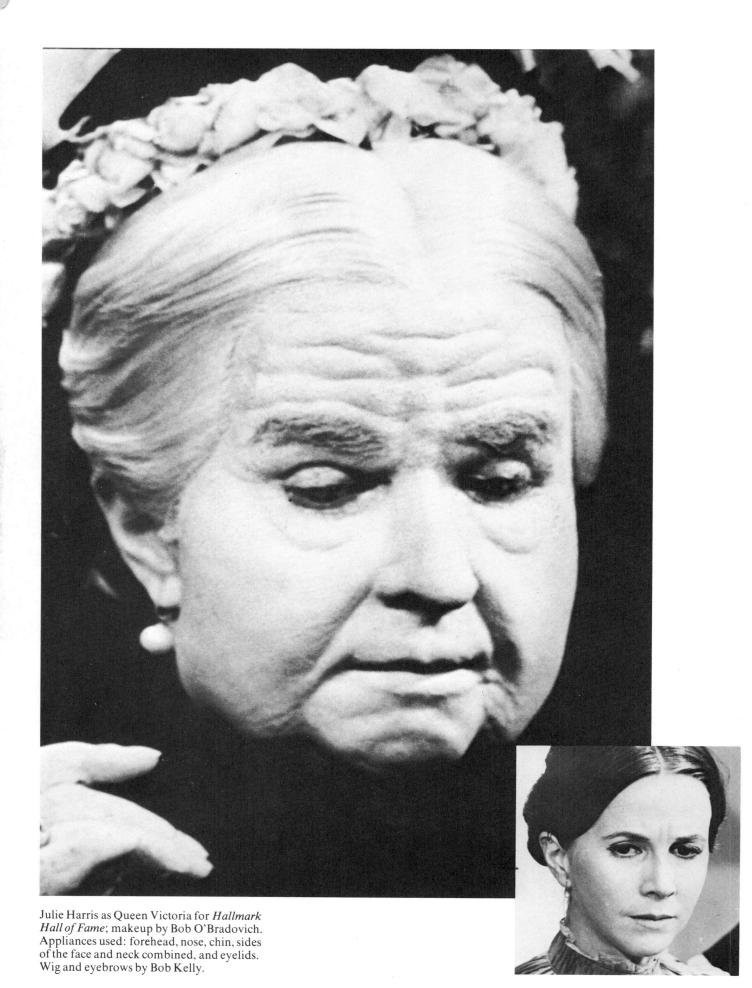

Julie Harris as Queen Victoria for *Hallmark Hall of Fame*; makeup by Bob O'Bradovich. Appliances used: forehead, nose, chin, sides of the face and neck combined, and eyelids. Wig and eyebrows by Bob Kelly.

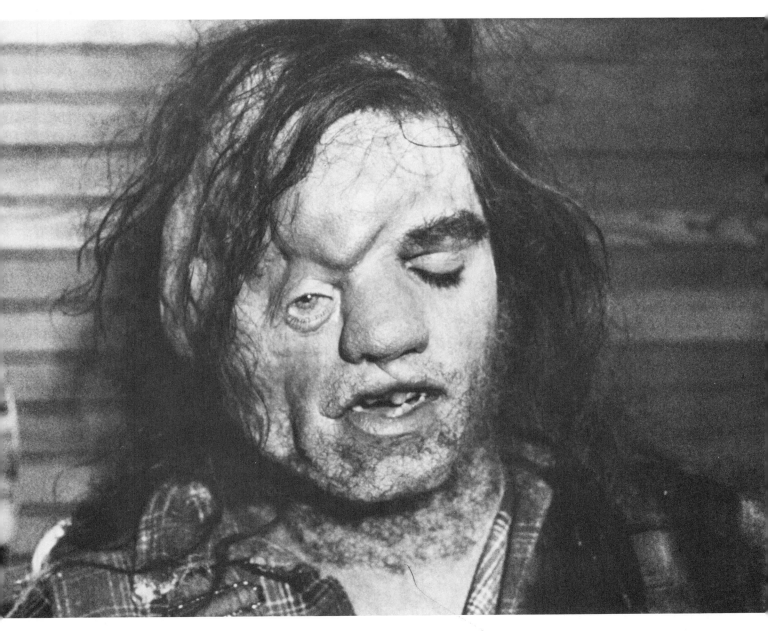

Warrington Gillette as Jason (above) and Tom McBride as Mark (right) in *Friday the 13th, Part II*; makeup by Carl Fullerton. Appliances used on Mr. Gillette on one side of the face only: top of the head, nose, side of the face, upper and lower lips, upper and lower teeth. Beard and eyebrows of yak hair were hand laid. The appliance used on Mr. McBride begins at the forehead and passes over the nose, nostrils, and upper lip and chin. Eyebrows laid by hand.

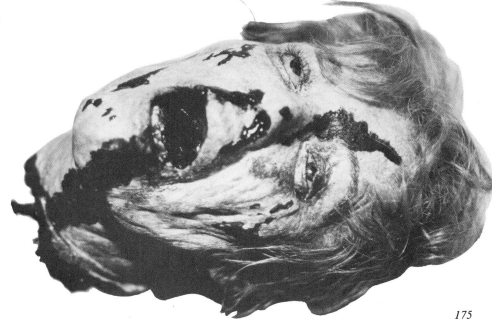

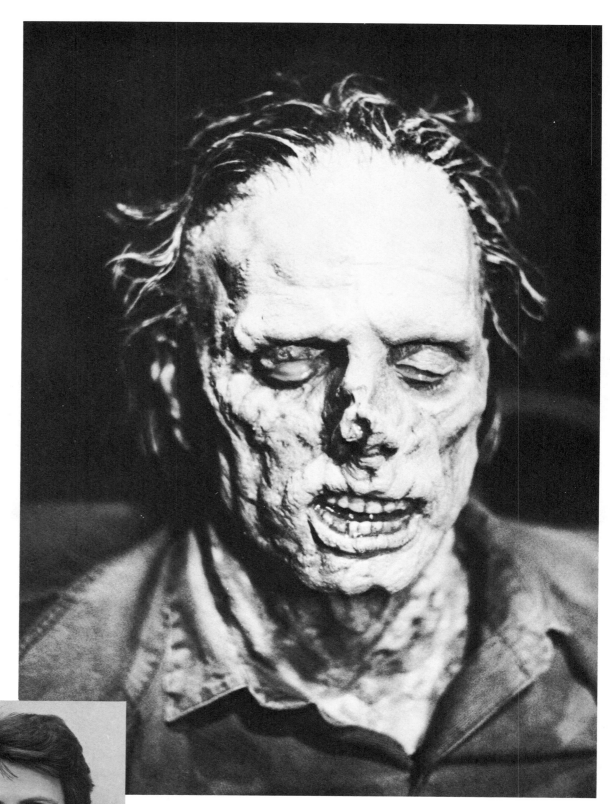

Kevin Haney used a series of foam-latex appliances to effect the transformation of actor Robert Burton on the NBC-TV show *Texas*. The final stage, shown here, is a dummy polyester resin head made from Burton's life mask. The hair was laid by hand and matted down with KY Jelly. The teeth were glossed with epoxy; the eyes were made of a mixture of epoxy and Cab-o-Sil.

APPENDIX

SOURCES OF MATERIALS

The following firms are sources of general makeup supplies:

Alcone Co. (formerly Para-
    mount Theatrical Supplies)
575 Eighth Avenue
New York, NY 10018
(212) 594-3980

Bob Kelly Cosmetics and
    Bob Kelly Wig Creation
151 West 46th Street
New York, NY 10036
(212) 819-0030

Leichner
599 Eleventh Avenue
New York, NY 10036
(212) 246-5443

Mehron, Inc.
250 West 40th Street
New York, NY 10018
(212) 997-1011

Ben Nye, Inc.
11571 Santa Monica Boulevard
Los Angeles, CA 90025
(213) 478-1558

Research Council of Makeup
    Artists (RCMA)
52 New Spaulding Street
Lowell, MA 01851
(617) 459-9864

M. Stein Cosmetics Co.
430 Broome Street
New York, NY 10013
(212) 226-2430

Note: Some of the following materials, including alcohol, acetone, 355 Adhesive, liquid latex, cap material, sealer, isopropyl myristate, spirit gum, spirt gum remover, MEK, DOP, and methyl chloride, can produce fumes, are harsh on the skin, and could produce allergic reactions. The sensitivity of the subject's skin should be taken into consideration when any of these materials is used, and all should be handled with care.

Acetone A clear liquid used to dissolve spirit gum, cap material, and sealer and to apply Celastic. It is harsh and flammable and so should be used carefully. Available at drugstores.

Acrylic Hygel A milky-white acrylic, used by artists as a transparentizing medium. It can be thinned with water and mixed with other colors. Here it is used to fix defective foam pieces as well as to repair thin edges of appliances. Available at art-supply stores; manufactured by M. Grumbacher, Inc., 460 West 34th Street, New York, NY 10001.

Acrylic Matte Medium An acrylic manufactured by Liquitex that can be brushed or stippled over and at the edges of bald caps. Available at art-supply stores.

Acrylic Paints Paints in all shades. When mixed with latex they create a permanent color that can be used over latex or foam-rubber pieces, or on any other area where rubber mask grease might rub off. In fact, they could be used instead of rubber mask grease anywhere. Available at art-supply stores.

Alcohol Isopropyl alcohol (90 percent) is used to dissolve spirit gum and to clean brushes and gummed laces on ready-made beards, wigs, and mustaches. Available at drugstores.

Alginate A powder known as Prosthetic Grade Cream which when mixed with water creates a paste that is used to cast faces, hands, teeth, and the entire body. Available from Teledyne Dental, Getz Apatow Division, 1550 Green Leaf Avenue, Elk Grove Village, IL 60007, (312) 593-3334.

Bald Cap A plastic or latex cap that covers the hair completely.

Latex caps are used mostly on stage, where with proper care they can be used for several performances. Available from Alcone, Mehron, Nye, and Stein.

Plastic bald caps are thinner. Unlike latex caps, the edges of plastic caps can be dissolved with acetone so that the edges are undetectable. They are used primarily in film and television. Available from Kelly and from John Chambers Studio, 330

South Myers, Burbank, CA 95106, (213) 846-0579, in three sizes: small, medium, and large.

Beaker A stainless-steel vessel about 6 inches (15 cm) in diameter and 8 inches (20 cm) high, the size for batches of foam latex recommended by manufacturers (see page 99). Larger sizes are available if needed. Available at hospital- and laboratory-supply houses.

Beaker of Water A plastic or glass beaker capable of holding at least 1,200 ml of water; it is best to use one that shows both milliliters and ounces. Available at laboratory- and photography-supply houses.

Brushes Artist's brushes have hairs made of different materials, such as sable or synthetics, and of different lengths, and they range in size from ⅛ to ½ inch (3 to 13 mm) wide. They are used to apply lipstick, cap material, and petroleum jelly, and for shading and blending. The choice of material, size, and quantity is up to you. All are available at art-supply stores, Alcone, Kelly, Nye, and Stein. Bent brushes (see page 112) are made by bending a regular brush with the hands or pliers.

Burlap Fabric used to reinforce molds. The best kind is loosely woven, which allows better penetration of the plaster into its fibers. Available at fabric stores.

B-11 See *Plaster.*

Butterfly Tweezers Tweezers with delicate, bent ends, used to hold prosthetic pieces during gluing (see page 112). Available from Rodnax Co., P.O. Box 6141, Vailsburg Station, Newark, NJ 07106.

Cab-o-Sil A thickening agent (amorphous fumed silica), used to prepare the first layer of PMC-724 when making a rubber negative mold (see page 164). Available from Cabot Corp., 125 High Street, Boston, MA 02110.

Dick Smith suggests: "Plastic Adhesive 355 can be matted to make an excellent glue for 'chopped-hair' beards. Use one teaspoon or more of Cab-o-Sil per ounce of 355. Moisten the Cab-o-Sil before mixing it in with trichloroethane." You can also mix Cab-o-Sil with regular spirit gum to get a matte finish.

Calipers An instrument for measuring, used to compare the sizes of the head and face or parts thereof with the sizes of the molds. Available at art-supply stores.

Cap Material A substance used to make plastic bald caps, to create scars, and to protect modeled clay pieces. It prevents modeled pieces from sticking to the nega-

tive molds. To make it, use four parts acetone (800 grams), four parts methyl-ethyl-ketone (MEK, 800 grams), one part VYNS (200 grams), and one-half part dioctyl phthalate (DOP, 100 grams). Pour all the ingredients into a bottle and shake or stir until the VYNS dissolves. It is then ready to be used. Cap material can be thinned with acetone.

Celastic A colloid-treated fabric like soft cardboard. When soaked in acetone, it becomes soft and can be used to reinforce molds (see page 31) or to hold seams and cracked areas together. Available at Alcone and art-supply stores.

Cellophane Paper A transparent paper that is used over clay models to create soft, natural-looking textures (see page 59). Available at art-supply stores.

Charlie Schram See *Foam Latex.*

Cheesecloth A loosely woven fabric used to strain liquid latex when it gets old and lumpy. When mixed with plaster, it can be used as a reinforcement. Available at fabric stores.

Clay See *Modeling Clay.*

Clear Lacquer Lacquer used over fresh molds as a separator for R and D foam. Available at art-supply stores.

Comb Used to pull the subject's hair out of the way.

Cotton Used to clean the last remaining modeling clay off the life mask (see page 88).

Cradle Used to hold the life mask of the full face. See page 19.

Dental Impression Plates Plates shaped to fit the mouth, used to take the impression of upper and lower teeth (see page 138). Available at dental-supply houses.

Denture Adhesive Adhesive used to hold the outer shell and inner section of the life mask together (see page 19). Available at drugstores.

DOP (Dioctyl Phthalate) A component of cap material. Available from Monsanto Chemical Co., St. Louis, MO, (800) 325-4336. (Note: DOP is harsh on the skin and has very strong fumes; use it with caution. Santicizer 160 or DBP—dibutyl phthalate—both of which are also available from Monsanto, could be substituted.)

Drills Used to create escape holes and keys in plaster molds; electric or hand drills can be used. Available at hardware stores.

Duo Surgical Adhesive Latex used to apply artificial lashes and to stipple over bald caps and all other latex and foam-latex appliances. Available at Di Lonardo and Rogg, 11 East 17th Street, New York, NY 10003, (212) 255-6120, and distributed by Narclif Thayer. Inc., Tuckahoe, NY 10707.

Face Mask Used when chemicals that produce harsh fumes are being used. Aseptex face masks are available from 3M Company, St. Paul, MN 55144, and at dental-supply houses.

Foam Latex The main ingredient of foam-rubber prosthetic appliances. R and D foam is what has been used in this book; it is available from R and D Latex Corp., 5901 Telegraph Road, Commerce, CA 90040, (213) 724-6161. George Bau's foam (see page 110) is available under the name of Charlie Schram from Windsor Hills Makeup Lab, 5226 Maymont Drive, Los Angeles, CA 90043, (213) AX1-5891.

Foam-Rubber Sponge A sponge used to apply basic foundation as well as rubber mask grease. Available at Kelly or from U.S. Rubber, 4402 11th Street, Long Island City, NY 11101, (212) 937-6800. Ask for pure poly foam, 36 by 96.

George Bau's Foam See *Foam Latex*.

Hair Brush Used to brush the subject's hair out of the way when the alginate life mask is being made.

Hair Clips Used to hold the alginate and shell together (see page 19).

Hair Whitener Whitener in blue, yellow, and off white, available in stick form at Alcone and Kelly; in liquid form at Alcone, Leichner, Nye, and Stein.

Hair Dryer Used to dry liquid latex over prosthetic pieces.

Hexane Suggested for mixing with Plastic Adhesive 355 (in equal parts). Available at Price-Driscoll Corp., 75 Milbar Boulevard, Farmingdale, NY 11735, (516) 249-4200.

Indelible Pencil Used to mark the subject's hairline over the bald cap before the life mask is cast (see page 15). Available at art-supply stores.

Isopropyl Myristate An ingredient of spirit gum removers. Can be used instead of alcohol or acetone to remove prosthetic pieces and bald caps. Available from City Chemical Corp., 132 West 22nd Street, New York, NY 10001, (212) 929-2723.

Japanese Brushes Watercolor brushes with bamboo handles and soft, pointed bristles. Not good for application of makeup, highlights, or shadows. Used to paint the first couple of layers of plaster inside the negative of the subject's life mask and over the modeled pieces. Also used to brush liquid latex inside a plaster or rubber mold to get the positive. Available at art-supply stores.

Lining Colors Colors in light and dark shades used to add shading, highlights, and general coloring to faces. Available at Alcone, Kelly, Leichner, Nye, and Stein.

Liquid Latex Used for aging and as coverage for foam-latex appliances and bald caps. Available at Alcone, Kelly, Nye, and Stein in small quantities. In large quantities it must be ordered through Major Chemical and Latex, Boston, MA (ask for prevulcanized latex IV-10); from General Latex, 666 Main Street, Cambridge, MA 02139; or from RCMA.

In its natural form latex can be ordered from Polymer Chemical Co., 131 Barron Drive, Cincinnati, OH 45215, (513) 771-6324. It is so thick that it must be spooned out of the drum, but it can be thinned with regular latex. Store it in a tightly closed container.

Liquid Green Soap Used to protect brushes before they are dipped in latex. Available at drugstores.

Log Book Any kind of notebook suitable for keeping records of all formulas, procedures, errors, and discoveries.

Makeup Remover A substance that removes makeup and spirit gum. If stippled over foam latex it creates swelling. Available at Kelly. Other types of makeup remover are available from Leichner, Mehron, Nye, and Stein.

Marking Pen Used to mark the bald cap or molds.

Masking Tape Used to tape down the plastic drop sheet covering the subject during casting of the life mask and to hold rubber-matting circles in place when molds are being made.

Measuring Cups Used to measure alginate, plaster, water, etc.

Measuring Stick A chopstick, swizzle stick, or similar stick marked at intervals, used to check the height of foam latex.

MEK (Methyl-Ethyl-Ketone) A component of cap material. Available at City Chemical Corp., 132 West 22nd Street, New York, NY 10001, (212) 929-2723.

Methylene Chloride A solvent used to clean cap material from clay models. Distributed by City Chemical Corp. (address above).

Mixer Used to mix foam latex. Professional mixers (see page 99) are available at laboratory-supply houses; a Sunbeam or other brand of electric mixer is available at hardware and department stores.

Modeling Clay Plastilina comes in white and gray green, in soft no. 1, medium no. 2, firm no. 3, and very hard no. 4 (see page 59). For larger models, Roma Plastilina is softer, has more oil, and dissolves more easily with alcohol. Available at art-supply stores and sculpture houses.

Modeling Tools Tools for sculpting made of wood, wire, and plastic in all shapes and sizes (see page 59). Available at art-supply stores and sculpture houses.

Muslin Towels Towels perforated all over, used to reinforce latex duplicates made with PMC-724. The perforations allow the latex to pass through and stick on both sides, which newsprint and paper towels won't do. Handi-Wipes can be used as well; available in supermarkets.

Nu-Gel Material used to cast teeth (see page 139). Available at dental-supply houses.

Old Age Stipple A makeup substance used to simulate old skin. The following is a basic formula for old age stipple, suggested by Dick Smith, which can be used instead of liquid latex:

Place 90 grams of Schram Foam Latex Base in an 8-ounce paper cup. This is a high-solid, creamed, natural latex with no fillers; consequently, it gives good texture and resists moisture pickup when dry. Mix together in another paper cup: 10 grams of talc U.S.P., 6 grams of pulverized CTV-5W Pancake, and 1 teaspoon plain Knox gelatin. Stir 3 tablespoons of very hot water into the powders, one at a time, until they are dissolved. Slowly, stir the solution into the latex. Pour this mixture into 2- or 3-ounce glass jars. Put the open jars into a hot-water bath for 10 minutes to ensure gelatin dispersal. Stir occasionally. This formula makes about 6 ounces. Cap and store in the refrigerator.

To use, heat a jar in a hot-water bath until the stipple becomes liquid.

This formula can be used without a rubber mask grease base. To remove powder from the stipple and to make it transparent, rub on a light film of castor oil and wipe it off; then add shadow and texture colors.

The 5W Pancake in the formula makes a color that matches average skin. Darker or lighter shades may be used instead.

If a stipple film comes loose in certain facial areas, paint them with a silicon adhesive. Powder the adhesive and then apply the stipple. Remove with soap and warm water.

Old age stipple works best if the subject has very pliable skin. After the formula is stippled over the stretched skin, it is dried, powdered, and the skin is let go. Stretching the skin horizontally makes vertical wrinkles, and stretching it vertically makes horizontal wrinkles.

Oven At first you can use your oven at home. For later work, however, a professional oven will be necessary (see page 99). Available at laboratory-supply houses.

Paper Cups Used to measure small amounts of ingredients such as jelling agent, curing paste, etc. One- and 3-ounce sizes are available from Edmund Scientific Co., 1980 Edscorp Building, Barrington, NJ 08007, (609) 547-8900. Or use plastic Dixie cups from Dixie Paper Co., Inc., 19 Avenue C, New York, NY 10009, (212) 228-6030.

Plaster Material used to make molds.
Plaster of Paris sets very quickly, but it is very soft and not durable, and it will not make accurate molds. Good only for brush-in latex.
White Hydrocal is fast-setting; it is not ideal for foam latex because the latex will stick to it. It can be used to make an original positive or for brush-in latex. It is not good for baking.
Ultracal 30 is much better for foam-latex molds. It sets slowly and stands up to the heat of the oven.
B-11 Hydrocal is slow-setting, fairly durable, and ideal for foam-latex molds.
Dental stone is very hard, accurate, and can be used to make foam-latex molds, but it does not stand up to baking any longer than B-11 and is very expensive.
Plaster is available from U.S. Gypsum Co.—check with the distributor in your area—and from Earth Materials, 588 Myrtle Avenue, Brooklyn, NY 11205, (212) 789-0782.

Plaster Bandage Gauze bandages impregnated with plaster. When wet and applied to alginate they create a hard shell. The best kind is made by Johnson & Johnson. It sets faster if submerged in water at 70° F. (21° C.) containing about 3 tablespoons of salt per pint. Available at Caligor Physicians and Hospital Supply Corp., 1226 Lexington Avenue, New York, NY 10028, (212) 369-6000. Or you can get Gypsona II plaster bandages, which are extrafast-setting, from Cheston, a division of National Development Corp., Dayville, CT 06241.

Petroleum Jelly Used as a separating agent over plaster. Available at drugstores.

Plastic Adhesive 355 Used instead of spirit gum to glue bald caps. 355 Medical Adhesive is available from Dow Corning Corp., Midland, MI 48640, (517) 496-4874; it is quite expensive. You can get it in small jars from RCMA as Prosthetic Adhesive, or

Kelly under the name Plastic Adhesive.
Dick Smith makes this suggestion: "Paint all the inside border areas of the cap, dry, and powder. Dust off the powder, put the cap on the subject's head, lift the edge, brush adhesive on the skin, wait a few seconds for it to dry, and press the cap edge down. Adhesion is instant and strong.
"In place of spirit gum, a diluted 355—one part 355 and one part hexane—can be used. This is a thin mixture with more strength than gum and slower-drying than pure 355. Where a stronger adhesive is needed, such as around the mouth, first apply a layer of 355, dry it, powder it; then position the appliance and apply the 355-hexane mixture over the powdered 355. The powdered adhesive will combine with the diluted 355 and give great strength. If you need even greater adhesion, also coat, dry, and powder the underside of the appliance with 355 before application."

Plastic Containers Used to cast ears (see page 148).

Plastilina See *Modeling Clay*.

Plexiglas Used as a base under molds or, when cut specially, to make square molds.

Pliers Used to cut and bend wire cloth to be used as reinforcement in molds.

Polyester Parfilm Used to spray inside solidified alginate before pouring the plaster to get the positive. Available at Price-Driscoll Corp., 75 Milbar Boulevard, Farmingdale, NY 11735, (516) 249-4200.

PMC-724 Used to make the negative of molds, the whole head or part of it. Available from Smooth-on, 1000 Valley Road, Gillette, NJ 07939, (201) 647-5800.

Powder, Translucent Used over makeup, rubber mask grease, and latex after it has dried. Available at Alcone, Kelly, Leichner, Mehron, Nye, and Stein.

Powder Puff Used to apply powder.

R and D Latex See *Foam Latex*.

Rasp Used to smooth out plaster molds. Available at hardware and art-supply stores.

Red A Creme Stick Used to stipple warm color over foam latex. Available at Kelly.

Red Rubber Sponge Used to texture clay models, to stipple color over foam latex, and for other uses. Available at Kelly, Leichner, and variety stores.

Router Bit A ¾-inch drill bit used to create round keys on molds with either a hand or an electric drill. Available at hardware stores.

Rubber Bowls Used to mix alginate or plaster.

Rubber Mask Grease Used especially to color foam latex and plastic caps. Available at Kelly and RCMA.
To make your own rubber mask grease, pulverize the right shade of Pancake makeup, add to it a few drops of castor oil, and mix until it is the right consistency. (It should not be too soft and oily; you will have problems with shine and inconsistent powdering.) Add to this a few drops of acetone, and mix thoroughly. Pour it into a jar, leave the lid off, and place the jar in a warm place so that the acetone will evaporate. Stir it often. Close it and place it in the refrigerator. Before using, allow it to come to room temperature.

Rubber Matting Flexible rubber in rolls, used in strips of different sizes to wrap around molds when making positives or negatives (see page 28). Available at hardware stores.

Rubber Stamps See page 61.

Ruler Used to measure plaster bandages.

Safety Razor Blade For general use in the laboratory.

Sandpaper Use to shape and smooth prosthetic teeth and for general use.

Scale Used to measure ingredients. Any kind that is accurate will do. We recommend a triple-beam balance that measures 2,610 grams, or a two-platform blance scale (see page 99). Available at Ohaus, Florham Park, NJ 07932.

Scissors For general uses.

Sealer A clear liquid used as a protection over wax or clay noses and chins. It dissolves in acetone. Available at Alcone, Kelly, Leichner, Mehron, and Nye.

Spatulas (Rubber and Metal) Used to mix alginate and colors, and to apply and blend wax. A valuable tool in the makeup kit.

Spirit Gum A liquid adhesive used to glue beards, wigs, bald caps, and prosthetic pieces. For television and film, matte spirit gum is preferable. It is advisable to leave the cap off the jar ahead of time to get it thick and gummy. Available at Alcone, Kelly, Leichner, Nye, and Stein.

Plastic Wrap Used to model over the life mask for accuracy of size and shape before transferring the clay pieces to their plaster positives (see page 73). Available at supermarkets.

Stipple Sponge A small black sponge used to press gently over wax or to stipple five o'clock shadow, or to color prosthetic pieces. Available at Alcone, Stein, and Kelly.

Stopwatch   Used to time the running of foam latex or the setting of alginate.

Surform Tool   Used to smooth plaster molds. Available at hardware stores.

Surgical Knife   Used to trim molds, cut unwanted bits and pieces from positives, and for general use. Available at surgical-supply houses.

Temporary Bridge Powder and **Temporary Bridge Resin**   Used to make teeth (see page 143). The generic name for these substances is methyl methacrylate. They must be self-curing. Available at dental-supply houses.

Tongue Depressor   Used to mix materials for casting a negative of the full head (see page 164). Available at medical-supply houses.

Toothbrush   Used to clean spirit gum from the laces of hairpieces and to apply whitener to hair.

Ultrocal 30   See *Plaster*.

Universal Tinting Colors   Colors that in proper combinations are used to color foam latex, in blue, white, green, red, yellow, raw sienna, burnt sienna, and raw umber. Universal Colorint is available from Benjamin Moore & Co., Montvale, NJ 07645; Tints-All, from Sheffield Bronze Paint Corp., Cleveland, OH 44119, and at art-supply stores.

VYNS   A plastic in powder form used to make cap material. Available from Union Carbide Chemical Co., 270 Park Avenue, New York, NY 10017, (212) 551-2345.

Water Clay   Can be used instead of modeling clay, not for modeling but in other areas where clay must be used, such as for reinforcement or walls.

Water Thermometer   Used to determine the temperature of the water when alginate is being used to cast a face. It must include at least the range between 60° and 80° F. 16° to 27° C.).

Wax   Used to build up a new nose or chin, cover eyebrows, or create scars. Available at Alcone, Kelly, Leichner, Nye, and Stein.

Weather and Humidity Reader   Used to check conditions that can affect alginate and foam.

Wire Cloth   Used to reinforce molds (see page 28). Available at hardware stores.

Wire Cutters   Used to cut wire cloth. Available at hardware stores.

Wooden Handle   Used for easy handling of positive molds (see page 22). Available at lumber yards.

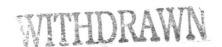

INDEX

Edited by Barbara Wood
Designed by Jay Anning
Graphic production by Ellen Greene
Photographs by Lee Baygan
Text set in 9-point Times Roman